The Revealin[g]
Uncensored,
Irreverent,
Detailed,
True Story!

PROTONS
VERSUS
PROSTATE CANCER
EXPOSED

Based on the
**Personal Experience of the Author,
Prostate Cancer Survivor**

Ron Nelson

Published by Little Pond Press
www.littlepondpress.com

PROTONS versus Prostate Cancer: EXPOSED
By Ron Nelson

ISBN: 978-0-9850823-0-7

**To the wonderful people at
The University of Florida Proton Therapy Institute**

for helping me find the humor

To Lucy

for everything else

Contents

Why I Wrote It / Why You Bought It 1

Fun with Prostate Cancer 7

Meet My PSA 9

Meet My Urologist 11

Take a Simple 60-Second Test 13

The Dreaded Biopsy 15

The Big News 19

Telling the Family 23

30 Days of Research 29

The Decision Matrix 33

Your Money or Your Life 37

Instructions from Florida Proton 41

Get Ready, Get Set 45

Go! Florida Phase 1 49

The Infamous Balloon 57

Phase 1: My First Tube 59

Phase 2: Poking & Prodding 63

Phase 2: Simulation 67

Southward, Ho! 75

Phase 3: Treatments 77

The 6 Stages of Balloonification 93

Between Treatments 99

Treatments with a Twist 109

The 3 P's: Pee, Poop, & Poke 113

Fringe Benefits 123

Lingering Questions 127

Tips for Future UFPTI Prostate Patients............................ 133

Proton Weenies 141

Appendix A: My Timeline... 143

Appendix B: Glossary of Terms 149

Acknowledgements... 157

About the Author 159

Why I Wrote It / Why You Bought It

I did not plan to write this book. In fact, I did not plan to get prostate cancer. And when I found out I had prostate cancer my reaction was not, "Hey, great, I think I'll write a book!"

But so many bizarre thoughts and convoluted ways of looking at my experience with prostate cancer, proton therapy, and life in general have popped into my head before, during, and after my diagnosis and treatment that I felt compelled to write them down so I wouldn't lose them, and to relieve the pressure building up inside my brain. There were just too many words crammed inside there, and I had to allow them to escape. Like acupuncture for the mind. So I wrote down everything—I've left *nothing* out—and then noticed there was enough of it for a pleasant little book.

Of the numerous books already written about prostate cancer and proton beam therapy in particular, this is probably the only one with no agenda other than my cerebral relief. In fact, I'm certain of it. As a consequence of that rather personal motive, you will find the information here more straightforward and less technical than most others on the subject, which might work quite nicely to round out your knowledge. When you finish reading it, you'll know everything I know. We'll be knowledge twins.

It's probably mostly a guy book. Men who have prostate cancer now or might get it later (hey, wait—that's *all* men) will certainly find it relevant. However, family members, loved ones, and especially wives who dare to venture into these rather personal pages will also find them enlightening. Guys are generally not adept at providing complete descriptions of what they're thinking, feeling, and experiencing, especially about something as personal as this. So I am hereby relieving them of that responsibility. We are pretty much in the same boat, so you guys can just hand a copy of this book to your loved one, saying, "Here you go, this'll tell you what you want to know," and then go have a beer.

But please remember, I did not set out to educate you, nor will I try to convince you of anything. I will simply do my best to tell you my complete, unabashed story and as a bonus, show you a good time. Be warned: you may have such a good time that even if you don't have cancer, you might wish you could have proton radiation anyway. It's that much fun. And when you've finished reading, you'll have a detailed understanding of what proton beam therapy for prostate cancer is really like.

I wrote this in a stream of consciousness. The contents simply spewed from my head as I mentally revisited the before, during, and after experience of being treated for prostate cancer at the University of Florida Proton Therapy Institute in Jacksonville. As you read, it will enhance your experience if you try to mentally hear my words in the voice of Walter Cronkite or Tom Brokaw. It will make it seem more important than it actually is, while also making it sound extremely professional. Be sure to swallow your L's if you choose Brokaw. If you're a lot younger than I am and have never heard of Cronkite or Brokaw, you are welcome to use Jon Stewart's voice in your head, as long as he adds credibility to my words. Actually, just go ahead and pick any voice you want. It's your head.

Also keep in mind that I did no research for this book, and it contains no intentionally useful information. I promise. The useful stuff is in Bob Marckini's terrific book on this subject: You Can Beat Prostate Cancer. It's based on his careful, thorough research and personal experience with proton treatment at Loma Linda University in California. If you have prostate cancer you should certainly read it before deciding how to treat your cancer. Please. Then after you complete proton radiation therapy (I'm making no assumptions here, just saying …), read this one for a pleasant, lighthearted stroll down memory lane with me. Or read mine first, and then his. I don't really care.

Now, please don't conclude or assume that Loma Linda specifically attracts, is more appropriate for, or somehow produces thoughtful, intelligent guys like Marckini, whereas Florida Proton just attracts guys like me. That would be unfair, and I am actually a very smart fellow, almost as smart as Marckini. It's just that he got his cancer before I did (not particularly fair), and then he wrote his landmark book and became famous, and yes, even a legend in his own time. Fine. Still, I'm a big enough man to admit we certainly don't need another book like his—he did a first-rate job. Writing a

Marckini knockoff book would add nothing to protons-for-prostate lore. It would be like some unknown little rock and roll band re-recording a Beatles hit, playing the song just like the Beatles played it, maybe even playing it well. But who needs that? If it was done right in the first place, leave it alone. It's done. So all that's left now for me is, well ... this.

For the record, my wonderful wife Lucy disagrees about the usefulness of this book. She thinks you will indeed find helpful information in my little story, but even if she is right (and she usually is right, just probably not this time), I absolutely categorically deny any forethought or intention of usefulness. If it turns out to be useful, it's a total accident and a lucky fluke. My purpose is to tell you *all* the details of what happened to me, what I thought about it, and how I felt. I suppose that in so doing, answers to questions left unanswered in other books might be found here. Oops! There. I've agreed with Lucy again. It might be useful, after all. But still, that was not my original intention.

On a loftier level, I could tell you I hope this book will be a vehicle for sharing my experience, helping others, becoming famous, making lots of money, becoming more philanthropic, hosting a radio show, giving commencement addresses, and eventually becoming a senator from my state or maybe the Surgeon General. Actually, all of the above are true. And why not? Other people have exploited the circumstances of their lives for comparable reasons, and so can I, by golly. And so far things are going very well. You bought a copy (or are planning to).

And why did you buy a copy? Aside from the obvious irresistible allure and promise of excitement from any book on prostate cancer, you will almost certainly fall into at least one of the following groups:

1. You have been diagnosed with prostate cancer.
2. You have been diagnosed with *prostrate* cancer.
3. You are concerned that you may later be diagnosed with #1 or #2.
4. You have already completed treatment for #1 or #2.
5. You know someone in one of the first four groups above.
6. You suspect you might someday meet someone in one of the first four groups above.

7. You suspect you have already met someone in one of the first four groups above, but don't know who it is.
8. You are pretty sure you know someone who knows someone in one of the first four groups.
9. You have an Amazon.com gift card collecting dust, and this book was an easy convenient way to use it.

I am most notably in group #4, but also in groups #5–8. I was diagnosed with prostate cancer in late 2010 and completed proton radiation therapy at the University of Florida Proton Therapy Institute (UFPTI) in March 2011, just a few months ago as I write. My perspective in this book will be from that vantage, and just so you know, I am totally pleased with the treatment I received and at least so far, the result. It was a most entertaining experience (more on that later).

CAVEAT EMPTOR

I want to be emphatically clear that it is not my intention to provide medical advice of any kind to anyone in any circumstance, and you would have to read way between the lines of this book to find anything that seems even a little like any kind of advice, especially the medical variety.

Actually, I do have one piece of advice for those yet to be treated: If you want indispensable information, read Bob Marckini's book. It's excellent. I already said that.

I also have a challenge for anybody who had a radical prostatectomy (open surgery, laparoscopic surgery, robotic surgery), cryosurgery, high intensity focused ultrasound (HIFU), brachytherapy (seed implants), intensity modulated radiation therapy (IMRT: photon/X-ray radiation), etc. If you can find sufficient material to write a "fun" book about your experience, please write it and let me know, as I have an Amazon.com gift card saved for that purpose.

And of course, for the sake of due diligence I must remind you that the views (if any) expressed in this book are mine alone, possibly shared by no one else on the planet (except maybe a few other prostate cancer patients), and certainly in no way imaginable represent the formal opinions of the professionals at the University of Florida Proton Therapy Institute. Informally, who knows.

Finally, most names have been changed to protect the competent.

Fun with Prostate Cancer

How exactly do you have fun with something as unpleasant as prostate cancer? Well, I have been there, done that, and you know, it is what it is, but it is also what you make it. I'm a glass-half-full kind of guy, so for me it was an amazing, unforgettable, and in many ways surprisingly positive experience. It also was, and continues to be somewhat surreal, and every day it strikes me as a bizarre characterization that I am "fighting my courageous battle with cancer," as people so often say with dour seriousness. I find that funny.

I'm not courageous, and I'm not fighting. I just get up every day, enjoy some coffee, pet my dog Baxter, go to work (I'm an I.T. guy for the county), come home, eat, exercise, maybe Skype my mother, play a little guitar, eat, watch some TV (Netflix, not live TV), eat, read my Kindle, explore the Internet, and enjoy the privilege and pleasure of spending my life with my awesome wife Lucy in every way I possibly can, which thankfully still includes first, second, and third bases, and yes, home runs, too (weekends and some Wednesdays).

I'm a lucky guy, and I don't spend much time thinking about cancer. But to be sure, my life has changed. I see things differently and my focus has shifted, and a lot more of it makes me laugh. There is so much humor in "my journey" (another phrase that makes me laugh) that I wanted to share my unique perspective, inviting you into my head (tread carefully there) to travel from the starting gate to the finish line with me. Maybe a smile will help lighten your load or that of someone you love.

I was lucky enough to be diagnosed at an early stage, and fortunate enough to be treated by the amazing people in Jacksonville. If you can complete the UFPTI program without looking back fondly and with humor, then your glass is probably half empty. In that case, I suggest flipping your glass over so it will be half full. Try it. Life is much more fun that way, even with prostate cancer.

Now, before I begin my story, I want you to be really excited about having this book, and thanks to watching a little bit of daytime

TV, I know exactly how to make that happen. Just follow these instructions:

1. Ask for assistance from the most animated person you know.
2. Put this book underneath the chair you're sitting in.
3. Ask your assistant to stand in front of you and recite the following with great energy, excitement, and authority while wildly waving his/her arms:

> *As you know, Ron Nelson's national runaway bestseller, his shockingly frank exposé on proton therapy for prostate cancer, has taken the nation by storm, and guess what: there is a copy for everyone under your chair RIGHT NOW!!!*

4. You should immediately stand up and start loudly screaming "YAY" while clapping your hands with great energy. Use whatever fantasy you need to make it seem real.

Trust me, this works. I've seen it on Oprah and other daytime shows and the excitement generated by this simple routine can send shivers down your spine even as a mere viewer, let alone as the one in the chair. It works even better with several participants, so I suggest having a Protons Exposed party (or maybe just call it Fun with Prostate Cancer), placing copies of this book under every participant's chair before completing the above steps.

So now that the thrill is on, settle back in your easy chair, relax, and prepare for an exciting and unforgettable voyage into the wacky world of prostate cancer. I hope it makes you smile. And remember, I'm not making this up.

Here is the story of my *journey*, fighting my *courageous battle* with cancer. Go me!

Meet My PSA

I had no idea what a PSA was until my primary physician, whom I'll call Dr. Perry, pointed out matter-of-factly that mine was a little high, just outside of normal. My reaction was the usual "So what, I feel fine" one that I use every time he identifies yet another slightly out of whack number. He is meticulous about finding the numbers that are just off the mark, and then he likes to tweak them with pills as soon as I'm willing. For example, he has successfully tweaked my cholesterol and triglycerides with a tiny round brown pill and an oval white one the size of a small suppository. I have started a nice little collection, similar to my Nana's pill lineup I remember marveling at as a young boy. I can still picture her foot-long string of pills, capsules, and tablets of every shape and color lined up on her kitchen counter as she scratched her balding head, puzzling over which ones to swallow just then. At the time I thought it was hysterical. Now I have started my own lineup.

So, my PSA was a little high, around 4. Okay, so "What's a PSA and why should I care?" I asked Dr. Perry. It turns out that the PSA is a prostate-specific antigen. Well, that explains everything, except I had no idea what the prostate did, or what an antigen was. However, I could certainly detect Dr. Perry's genuine concern, so I pursued this further and he gave me one of his trademark shoulder-shrugs, explaining that the prostate is a male gland *blah blah blah blah blah ...* and it is not unusual for a *man my age* to have a slightly elevated PSA due to a slightly enlarged prostate, also common for *men my age*. Now, my mother is 88, which is old, and I am merely her son—her little boy—so how can a phrase like "men my age" apply to me? I am *lots* younger than my mother! I am a young man. Just look inside my head and you'll see. My mother (as I said) is old (though incredibly vibrant, smart, and active). She is a *woman her age*. I am not a *man my age*. But, this characterization seemed to placate Dr. Perry to some degree, and because of it he was willing to suggest we merely keep an eye on the PSA level. No pills or other tweaks yet. Okey dokey.

Over the next 18 months and several blood tests, we indeed watched my PSA rise, and rise, and rise again. Not to terrifying

4-alarm fire heights, but a steady ascent into the 4–5 range. Dr. Perry was concerned about the so-called acceleration, and apparently there was no little pill of any shape or color to adjust my PSA (darn). So I wondered, what now, Dr. Perry?

His next move was to refer me to a urologist for a consultation regarding my rising PSA. A *urologist!!!! What?????* I am not old enough to want, need, or have my own urologist! It would seem that I have not only accumulated my own potpourri of pills (there are now five), I must also expand my army of doctors to include not only my family doctor, dentist, ophthalmologist, dermatologist, ear-nose-throat guy, and gastroenterologist, but also my very own personal *urologist*. I must be either extremely healthy with this talented entourage, or in deep doo doo.

Meet My Urologist

As it turned out, I love my urologist. He is probably the most direct, forthright, and (most importantly) wry of my ever-growing tribe of excellent physicians. Kind of a country doctor who delivers news with a *shrug,*[1] and optionally *a chuckle* if he thinks you can handle it. Very laid back, matter-of-fact, smart, compassionate, "pee" doctor, as he calls himself. I'll call him Dr. Pee.

Within minutes of my first meeting with Dr. Pee, I was bent over receiving the pleasure of his personal variation of a DRE[2]: quick, and uneventful, completely absent of ceremony or fanfare. This was in marked contrast to the annual DRE Dr. Perry included as the climax event (oops, no pun intended) of my annual physical. Dr. Perry would ask me to disrobe, leave the room, return about ten minutes later (thinking, I suppose, that disrobing could be a complicated matter for a *man my age*), knock on the door, ask if I was ready, enter without looking directly at me, and snap on his rubber glove, lubricating it as he apologized and proclaimed he didn't like doing it any more than I liked receiving it ("it," I suppose, being his digit; I'm still not sure which one he uses). On the other hand (again, no pun intended), Dr. Pee's instructions were a simple, terse, "Drop your pants and bend over" and BAM—it was done. All things considered, I prefer that approach.

In fact (and this little factoid is chronologically out of sequence), there is at least one other DRE technique I experienced only once, in Florida. My oncologist (OMG, another member of my

---

[1] All my doctors seem to like the *shrug.* I wonder if they teach that in medical school.

[2] It occurs to me now that you might not know what DRE stands for, so here's a good scientific definition for you, just in case: it is a digital rectal examination. Unfortunately, "digital" does not refer to the technology of digitizing data or any of the sophisticated electronics associated with that; in this case, "digital" means using a finger. "Rectal" means via the butt hole. "Examination" means, more or less, exploration. A DRE provides the most convenient non-surgical access to the proximity of my beloved prostate. The doctor can indirectly feel the prostate and assess its condition. I had always suspected this was a multi-purpose portal, and I was right.

medical entourage) wanted to cop a feel himself. For him, I was on a table on my back, knees up, legs apart, and *woops*—there it is, now it's done. I'm pretty sure it was the right hand middle finger. Not that it matters. I'm also pretty sure I didn't deliver a baby, although I was properly poised.

Dr. Pee informed me that my prostate was a little big ("slightly enlarged"), but okay (he was kind enough to omit "for a man your age"). It was firm, with good elasticity, and nothing unusual (like a palpable tumor, a lump he could feel). He seemed pleased, and gave me a big ol' country doc smile. I smiled back. I was hoping for elasticity and I got it. Made my day. He opined that I probably did not have cancer (whew—first use of the "C" word), and if I was in agreement, we would just keep an eye on things for a while.

Come back in six months.

This time things went even quicker, and no DRE, which very much surprised but did not disappoint me. After all, he's that guy, right? That's what he does. He can have his way with me any time he wants, right? Anyway, that made my day. But just in case it was an oversight I said, "What? No DRE?" and he replied, "It won't be any different than last time, so why bother?" Cool!

But my PSA was up again, closer to 5 than 4. Still, he wasn't particularly worried, did not want to do a biopsy (OMG, a *biopsy*???) yet (*yet*????), and said:

Come back in six months.

And then my PSA had reached the high 5s (not the celebratory kind), and Dr. Pee was not so sure any more. Maybe we should consider a biopsy. But wait! There's one more option to consider first.

Take a Simple 60-Second Test

Dr. Pee described a relatively new urine test (remember, he's the self-proclaimed "pee" doctor) called a PCA3. It's quick and simple, and it predicts the likelihood a biopsy would be positive. Hmmmm, wouldn't that be the same as predicting I have …

Anyway, here's how it works: after a DRE, about the first ounce of urine is taken and tested for PCA3, which is only produced by cancerous cells. This is good information to have in addition to the PSA level. PSA can be ambiguous because it is produced by both cancerous and non-cancerous cells (as in age-related normal prostate enlargement, or prostatitis: infection of the prostate.) A PCA3 score of 35% or greater is considered positive and means, well, you know.

This all sounded too easy, so I asked:

Me: So, it's just a regular DRE, and then a urine sample?

Dr. Pee: Well (*shrug*), not exactly regular. The DRE is not quite as quick, and involves massaging the prostate into the bladder, 30 seconds on the right, then 30 on the left.

Me: Massaging? What exactly does that mean?

Dr. Pee: Well (*shrug*), I push the prostate up against the bladder with more, uh, more, well let's say, as compared with a regular DRE, it's might be just a little more, uh …

Me: Enthusiastic?

Dr. Pee: Right!!! Yeah! (*grin*) Enthusiastic. That's it (*hehehe*). Very clever. I like that! An enthusiastic, vigorous massage.

Me:	So, how will it feel (*thinking it almost sounds sort of relaxing*)?
Dr. Pee:	Well, of course you're going to want to pee. Badly, very badly, but don't worry, you won't be able to.
Me:	Well, that doesn't sound so bad. No anesthetic or anything? Just a feeling of wanting to pee for a minute? I think I can handle that.
Dr. Pee:	Right, but let me be clear. You will *really really really* want to pee, but only for that minute, and then you can. We need the first ounce.

He gave me some information about the PCA3 test to read, told me to decide if I wanted it, and if so, call him back to schedule the test. It certainly sounded better than a biopsy, so of course I went for it. Had it done six weeks later.

Here is how I remember it. During that one-minute massage I would have paid a million dollars, given up my first-born, and cut off my right arm if only he'd have let me pee. I have never, ever wanted to pee so badly in my life. Ever. Think about the most urgency you've ever felt, and multiply it by 100. Or by 1000. Whatever. This intense feeling was accompanied by sudden onset Tourette's Syndrome (from me, not the doctor). I immediately began spewing venomous language at an unprecedented rate and with amazing and somewhat surprising skill while he chuckled and enthusiastically massaged.

Then, what felt like six months later the "minute" was over and he said: "Okay, done. Take this cup into the bathroom and give me the first ounce. Take your time. No hurry." And ironically, after all that, I could barely get a stream started. I guess he had squished my urethra a little, maybe? Or left his digit behind? Anyway, it took a few minutes, but I finally did produce the prized golden ounce.

And off it went to the lab.

The Dreaded Biopsy

Four weeks later my PCA3 results came back positive. Mine was 50%, and over 35% is a go for a biopsy. So I did not dodge the biopsy bullet after all, but I did have the pleasure of the PCA3, a bonus not everyone experiences.

Courtesy of the PCA3 test, a biopsy was now deemed *likely to be positive*, so we scheduled it. I had this conversation with my urologist:

Dr. Pee:	Well (*shrug*), I think maybe we should go ahead and schedule a biopsy.
Me:	So exactly how does that work?
Dr. Pee:	Well, I go in through the rectum and take a dozen tissue samples and blah blah blah blah **needles** blah blah blah blah …
Me:	Whew! I'll have a general anesthetic for that, right?
Dr. Pee:	Well (*shrug*), it's usually done with a local.
Me:	Really? It doesn't sound much better than a colonoscopy, and my gastroenterologist used a general. Why not for a prostate biopsy?
Dr. Pee:	As a group, urologists are a generally meaner bunch than gastroenterologists (*grin*).
Me:	Okay, well, can I specifically request a general if I prefer one?
Dr. Pee:	Sure, you can request a general (*wink*).
Me:	Fine, consider this my request. Knock me out.
Dr. Pee:	So noted. Will do.

After scaring the poop out of me with the threat of not being given a general anesthetic, I later learned Dr. Pee routinely uses a general for prostate biopsies. Funny guy. I guess he needs to get his kicks somehow.

Come back in four weeks.

My wife drove me there as instructed, to enjoy the rare spectacle of me on my side with a variety of paraphernalia stuffed up my hiney while being televised on the nearby monitor, and to drive me home afterward, assuming she'd still want me after seeing me violated in such a bizarre manner. In her shoes, I might have quietly snuck out the door when no one was looking, leaving cab fare on the table.

Anyway, here's how it went. I had a late afternoon appointment with Dr. Pee. We arrived punctually, and then waited for a couple hours. Did I mention he is a laid back, country sort of doc? When he's consulting with you (meaning me) he is never rushed, takes *aaaaalllllllllllllll* the time in the world, tells lots of entertaining anecdotal stories, and would give the illusion that you (meaning me) are his only patient. This is great when you are with the doctor, but not so great when you are waiting as we were then. But I want to be perfectly clear (in case Dr. Pee is reading this) that I think this is a fair tradeoff. When necessary, I am willing to wait for my turn at a relaxed, fun, always informative consultation with my beloved pee doc.

So Lucy and I killed a couple hours reading in Dr. Pee's waiting room and roaming aimlessly around the building. I made frequent bathroom stops in order to make sure my bladder was empty during the procedure, so as to not embarrass myself. As it turned out, this only eliminated one of several options available to embarrass myself, and Lucy tells me I was successful at finding others. I am pretty skilled at that, yes indeed.

When it was finally my turn, we were ushered into the procedure room, which I can still picture clearly. We each sat in our respective chairs, and were soon greeted by Dr. Pee and his also somewhat wry nurse. She wordlessly handed me a big plastic syringe, and being a little slow on the uptake, I was confused.

Me: What should I do with this?

Nurse: Stick it in your mouth, toward the back.

Me: And then?

Nurse: Squirt and swallow.

Me: Ah.

It contained Versed in liquid oral form. I was reminded that this would cause me to have some problems with memory for the rest of the evening. As we waited for it to kick in, Dr. Pee took us for a stroll down memory lane, talking about the bizarre things some of his prior patients had done on the way home from a procedure involving Versed. In addition to killing time, this was intended to dissuade me and particularly Lucy from stopping at restaurants or otherwise appearing in public after my biopsy while still medicated with happy juice, even though I might possibly want to do so. I do not feel authorized to repeat those stories, but I encourage you to ask your urologist to share some Versed stories with you. They were most entertaining, and they are the last thing I even vaguely remember from that visit. I do not recall disrobing at all, but in hindsight (no pun there, right?) I am sure I must have at least partially undressed, and also probably somehow climbed up onto the operating table, and then off again. That Versed is good stuff.

Lucy was there the entire time, so I have a witness and feel confident that I did, in fact, have a biopsy. Although I suppose it is possible there was no real connection between what was happening in my derriere and what was being broadcast on the little TV Lucy was watching (remember the so-called moon landing staged for TV in the 60s?). Nevertheless, I chose to take that leap of faith and believe that the information resulting from this excursion into never-never-go-there-land was factual, rather than conspiratorial fiction. I trust Dr. Pee. Had no choice, really.

Lucy's job as Dr. Pee's deputy was to help keep me on my right side while on the table, facing the TV monitor. She could also see the monitor and the doctor, and reports that along with the ultrasound scope, needles were used as promised, and twelve little snips were made to remove the dozen samples. She says it was kind of cool, and I am happy she enjoyed it.

Because Versed so effectively and continuously wiped out my short-term memory during this visit, I'll have to tell you courtesy of Lucy's memory that I apparently did have a few questions during the procedure. How many samples would he take? Would he have a preliminary guess at the results? What could he see on the ultrasound image? Could we go out to eat afterward? How many samples would he take? Would he have a preliminary guess at the results? What could he see on the ultrasound image? Could we go out to eat afterward? How many samples would he take? Would he have a preliminary guess at the results? What could he see on the ultrasound image? Could we go out to eat afterward? How many samples would he take? Would he have a preliminary guess at the results? What could he see on the ultrasound image? Could we go out to eat afterward? And so on, never remembering the answers, looping the same questions throughout the procedure and hours afterward. It takes more than patients to be a doctor; it takes patience.

Apparently Dr. Pee tired of endlessly repeating answers to the same questions, and Lucy tired of this as well. So realizing my brain was unplugged anyway, they decided to amuse themselves by providing answers designed to entertain each other rather than to inform me, especially to the last question about going out to eat, which had already been addressed before I swallowed the Versed. So yes, we could go out to dinner, have a big steak and whatever else I wanted, the meal of my dreams. I could hardly wait! I have no idea how else they might have messed around with my mind, and I suppose I'd rather not know. As long as they had a wonderful time. That's what's really important.

My memory mechanism did not begin recording again until much later that night, long after the biopsy was over. Lucy graciously fielded a few questions from me on the drive home (see questions listed above), she told me. Thankfully, she did not open the passenger door and push me out while driving on the interstate, which might have been an understandable temptation. In any case, we made no stops, did not get the promised steak dinner, did not stop anywhere for food of any kind, did not stop for a quick game of paintball, and went straight home.

I am pleased to report (and thank Dr. Pee) that unlike too many biopsy horror stories I have since heard (mostly involving local anesthetic only), mine was a non-event for me. Lucy observed the procedure, and reported that I did well and seemed to suffer little *discomfort*. Don't you love that word?

Come back in a week.

The Big News

During the time between my biopsy and the consultation that followed, Lucy and I had already adjusted to the extreme likelihood that, given the escalating PSA and the positive PCA3, my biopsy would be positive. With that expectation, we sat down with Dr. Pee, and he did not disappoint us.

Dr. Pee: Well, I have good news and bad news.

Me: Okay.

Dr. Pee: The bad news is the biopsy was positive. The good news is that it's your *prostate*, not your lungs, liver, bones, blood, or pancreas. When it comes to the "C" word, it's the word that precedes it that counts.

Me: Okay.

Dr. Pee: So, we can talk about treatment options, any of which should work for your early stage. If you had one of the other varieties I'd probably be referring you to a mortician (*hahaha*), but I can give you lots of options, any of which should take care of what you have.

Me: Okay, so I have prostate cancer. What's next?

Dr. Pee was clearly going overboard to be sensitive to the anticipated extreme reaction people often have when learning they have cancer—any cancer. He seemed to be avoiding the word, and wanted to repeatedly stress that *prostate* cancer was different than all the others. Okay, I'm fine with that, I have the "good" kind of cancer (*woo hoo!*). Lucy and I just wanted to move on. So …

Dr. Pee: Well, you could continue to wait—active surveillance, as some call it—but at an early stage of disease, an otherwise healthy man your age with a long life expectancy probably wouldn't be wise to wait.

Wow! First time *a man your age* meant *young*! I was *only* sixty, a young man, as I pointed out earlier. So glad to see someone recognizing that, at last.

> Dr. Pee: There are lots of treatment options. You could throw a dart to pick one and it would likely cure your cancer …

Dr. Pee was now adjusting to the fact that we were okay with the "C" word, and were ready to move on.

> Dr. Pee: … but the side effects and quality of life issues differ, so you have to research the options carefully and decide which you are most comfortable with. They all have potential side effects that can affect quality of life.

This "quality of life" thing is something I wasn't perfectly clear about yet. But I did know it was sufficiently significant to justify its own acronym, QOL, so it must be important. I was listening carefully.

> Dr. Pee: Surgery is an option. I do surgery. There is traditional open surgery, laparoscopic surgery, and robotic surgery. All would remove the prostate, but I don't think surgery is the best option for you.

I have learned that coming from a urologist, this opinion is most extraordinary. Urologists are often surgeons (as is Dr. Pee), and surgeons often—maybe usually—recommend cutting. Surgeons cut. I have heard stories of urologists who summarily banished patients who had the audacity to choose another treatment modality, and here was my guy, telling me surgery might just be a bad idea for me. Quite a rarity, and a stroke of luck.

> Me: Why not surgery?

I was about to have my first mini-anatomy lesson. I hated anatomy and biology in high school, found it boring and irrelevant. It was relevant now, and I was still listening carefully.

Dr. Pee: Well, it's tricky. You see, the bladder sits right on top of the prostate, the rectum is right behind, it, the urethra runs through the middle of it, and the nerves for sexual function are all around it, so it's really hard to get to the prostate and (*shrug*) a lot can go wrong.

Me: Whoa.

Dr. Pee: It's the quality of life we're concerned about. Incontinence and impotence are the most troublesome possible side effects. Those are the risks with any approach to treating the prostate, and we like to try to avoid them.

Me: Yes, we certainly do.

Dr. Pee: Surgery would work, but you can also consider Brachytherapy (radioactive seeds), IMRT (photon radiation), a combination of seeds and photon, HIFU (ultrasound), cryosurgery, proton radiation, or watchful waiting. Probably not cryosurgery, HIFU is not done in the U.S. yet, and I don't think more waiting will be helpful.

As Lucy and I listened to Dr. Pee describe the pros and cons of each option, we detected a subtle nudge towards proton radiation, about which he admitted knowing relatively little.

Me: You seem to be strongly implying I should investigate proton. Am I misreading that?

Dr. Pee: No, that would be accurate.

Me: And why is that?

Dr. Pee: I hear the side effects may be fewer. Do the research and see what you think. I have another patient, an ex-CIA type of guy who

	researched this up the wazoo, and he completed proton therapy in Florida last March. I'll see if he'll agree to talk with you, if you want.
Me:	By all means. Thanks. So, how long before I should make a decision?
Dr. Pee:	No big rush, but start your research now and decide as soon as you can. Let me know.

I was not going to wait. No more active surveillance, watchful waiting, or diligent dawdling for me. Those phrases were starting to sound more like "innocent bystanding" or "wishful thinking," which amounted to doing nothing. It was time to take action to treat the cancer, and having made that decision, I could no longer regard time as my friend. I had to get moving.

And so began my courageous battle with cancer on October 21, 2010.

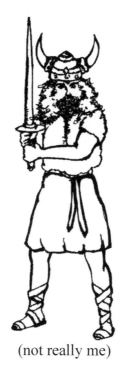

(not really me)

Telling the Family

Although Lucy and I were focused like a laser on research and resolution (R&R) of this prostate cancer annoyance, informing my mother, mother-in-law, daughters, close friends, and work associates was unavoidable and a delicate matter. While I felt confident this cancer thing would have a positive outcome, I shared Dr. Pee's concern of how people might react. I mean, one way or another I was going to announce I had cancer, and yeah, that sounds kind of bad.

So I mentally tried out various lines, such as:

> *Oh, by the way, I have cancer, but it's the* <u>*good*</u> *kind. YAY!*

Nah. Maybe this:

> *Now, sit down and don't be alarmed, this is not as bad as it might sound at first.*

Nope. How about:

> *Well, I have a health update for you. I'm going to be treated soon for prostate* *CANCER... CANCER... CANCER...*

I don't think so. Try this:

> *First, let me say that I'm going to be fine, just fine, so please don't worry, really.*

By that point the listener would no doubt be worried out of their skull, and may need treatment of their own. Here's a fun one:

> *Guess what disease has a better than 90 percent cure rate, which by the way I happen to have?*

Hmmm, that might be getting closer to the mark.

Of all the kinds of cancer, which one is your
personal favorite?

Sounds a little silly, but it would certainly get their attention.

After banging my head against the wall for a little too long, I finally decided to tell my four daughters all at once by email. At the risk of becoming dated before this book is even published, I'll go out on a limb and declare that email is one of several widely used electronic forms of communication, especially in their generation. Email would allow me to choose my words carefully, while giving each daughter time to digest the information in her own way, at her own pace. Then later we could have one-on-one conversations about it whenever they were ready.

I'm too lazy to do the exact age-calculation math right now, but they were all adults ranging from about 24 to 36 years old when I sent this to them in October 2010. Here is the exact message I sent, prior to having made a final decision about which kind of treatment I would choose:

Subject: My new health challenge

Hi, kids.

I am going to have to be treated for a relatively unaggressive, highly localized, early-detected case of prostate cancer, very common in men (1 in 6), and increasingly likely with age. Unless you are an older guy (hahaha) you might not know that cancer of the prostate when detected early is probably the least threatening variety, and highly treatable. So I am not worried and neither should you be worried. If the word "cancer" bothers you, remember that this is not liver cancer or pancreatic cancer or lung cancer or bone cancer or even breast cancer ... it is the best of the bunch: prostate cancer.

So there is nothing particularly pressing about this. Prostate cancer progresses very slowly, and mine is entirely localized within the prostate—no spreading. I have time to consider which treatment option I want, and there are many. This is really the challenging part, and I have been doing a lot of research. I could, but almost certainly will <u>not</u> have surgery (open, laparoscopic, or laparoscopic/robotic), cryosurgery, or *chemotherapy. I will probably have some form of radiation therapy, and I am very interested in proton radiation (as opposed to more traditional x-ray/photon radiation). I might also consider brachytherapy, which involves insertion of small radioactive seeds directly into the prostate.*

Whatever I choose, it will certainly be disruptive to my life and Lucy's both financially (even with insurance, already degraded thanks to recent legislation) and otherwise. Depending on the treatment, I might need to be out of town for possibly 4–8 weeks, miss work, etc. There will also be follow-ups, etc. I'm not looking forward to it, but it has to be done.

I expect to make a decision and have treatment within the next 6 months. Once I decide on a treatment I will tell Gramma Hecky and Mama Bailey. Until then, you (and your spouse) are the only ones who need to know, and I'd appreciate it if you kept it that way. If you feel anyone else should be included please check with me first—thanks.

If you want to join in and help me research the treatment options, I'll be glad to send you the key diagnostic information. You might be better at finding the relevant research than I am!

I decided to email rather than call you in order to let you all know at the same time, but feel free to call with any concerns, questions, or suggestions. I should be home after lunch tomorrow. I have to scrape the road in the morning, before too many leaves fall.

Love,
Daddy

That seemed to work pretty well. I received some quick email replies and then had extensive phone calls with all four girls. As expected, each reaction was very different and required a unique kind of conversation, but in the end I think everyone understood that in life's rear view mirror, this would in all likelihood be nothing more than a speed bump.

Somewhat later, I informed the thirty or so fine folks in the Information Technology Department of Richland County, South Carolina by email, too. These are my friends and coworkers, and I wanted them all in the loop. Here is my message to them, sent after I had decided that proton beam therapy was the best approach and the one I would pursue:

Subject: Health news

Fellow IT folks,

> *Rather than let you find out through the department grapevine, I want to tell you all directly that I have very early stage prostate cancer. Of the many effective treatment options, I have opted for proton beam radiation therapy at the University of Florida Proton Therapy Institute, the closest of only ten such facilities in the U.S. Cure rates with this technology are above 90%, so I feel very confident about a successful outcome.*

> *I will have to take a week off this month for tests and imaging before actual treatment can begin early next year. Then I'll be staying in Jacksonville for 8 weeks for treatment. Treatments are given Monday–Friday, and are brief and painless with minimal side effects. My expectation is to work from Jacksonville. Obviously I won't be able to conduct meetings during those weeks, but I can effectively keep up with email and other work in progress not requiring my physical presence, so I don't expect to be bored between treatments. Thank goodness for remote connections.*

> *While I don't think this needs to be a secret, I intend to inform those outside our department only when necessary and appropriate. If there's anything more you want to know about this, please stop by my office any time. I'd be glad to answer any questions.*

> *Ron*

This was also effective, and several people, men and women, stopped by to talk with me about prostate cancer and proton therapy. Many had no idea what a PSA was. Can you imagine that? So my email became an effective tool for spreading prostate cancer awareness among men and their wives with whom I work. I am now the resident authority, and a couple guys watching their PSA give me regular updates. My office is Prostate Cancer Central.

I told my mother (Hecky to the rest of the world) via a Skype video call. The visual part of a conversation was very important in conveying my optimism along with the raw information. She took it well enough—my cousin had survived prostate cancer five years earlier—but she didn't like it. After all, she's my mother. I'm glad she didn't like it. She's not supposed to like it. As I recall, I didn't especially like it, either.

My mother-in-law had her own style: short and to the point. So telling her was relatively easy, and face to face was best. With her, I was able to be blunt and direct. "Well, I have prostate cancer, but it's not going to be a problem. They can cure it." And that was that.

Telling the guys can be even easier. I told my brother-in-law and nephew in a few minutes while they were stacking firewood. "Hey, guys. Got prostate cancer. Darn. Going to Florida for a couple months to get rid of it." They said they were sorry to hear it, good luck, and keep them posted. No big deal. Back to stacking wood.

My 21-year-old niece, sweet girl, had a slightly different reaction: could she get prostate cancer, too? Just goes to show that we learn about some things in life only when necessary. Now she can rest comfortably that at least one type of cancer is absolutely off her list.

The bottom line is that there just isn't a foolproof way to break the news gently to anyone, and there is no single good way to tell everyone. But it had to be done, it was done, and no one had a heart attack when I told them. On the plus side (for me), I got a lot of sympathy in the process, which was very cool. This was my first glimpse at the substantial package of fringe benefits awaiting us as cancer victims (more on that in a later chapter).

One way or another, the challenge of informing your friends and family is unavoidable. You have to just bite the bullet, tell them somehow, and hope for the best. You can't keep it a secret. They deserve to know.

Feel free to use any of the above ideas if you think they'll be helpful in breaking the news to your loved ones, no royalties required.

30 Days of Research

So, other than curing the cancer—which thankfully seemed likely with any approach to treatment—quality of life was the goal and main focus of my research. Urinary incontinence? Fecal incontinence? Impotence? Yikes! Maybe I'll just take the cancer behind door #1.

I absolutely had to get this right. No do-overs. So I began spending all my available waking hours reading anything I could find about treatments and outcomes. Most of this research was on the Internet. What would we do without the web? Also, lots of worthwhile information came from my research-expert Ph.D. daughter Jessica, who pitched right in and found some excellent articles I would have missed. And of course, Bob Marckini's book was extremely helpful. I was on my way to becoming an authority on the treatment of prostate cancer.

I quickly became an avid student of a certain part of the male anatomy, commonly referred to as the pelvic area. What I learned is that this area involves some REALLY CRAPPY DESIGN! I mean, unless the idea is to make sure you can't get to the prostate (if necessary) without royally screwing up lots of other critical stuff. The bladder (for peeing) sits right on top. The rectum (for pooping), next door. The urethra (for pee and semen), directly through it. And the cavernous nerves (for erections) all around it. In an MRI of my prostate I am pretty sure I saw a notice reading, "WARNING: STAY BACK!" And that's your human anatomy lesson for the day.

So the question is, how can I stop or otherwise get rid of the cancer inside my prostate without messing up the valuable stuff I'm quite fond of all around it? Unfortunately, it just can't be done, at least not with today's technology. I'll just have to try to make my best educated guess at which treatment modality will minimize the collateral damage that will likely occur to some degree with them all.

Diagram of Author's Anatomy
(not actual size or scale)

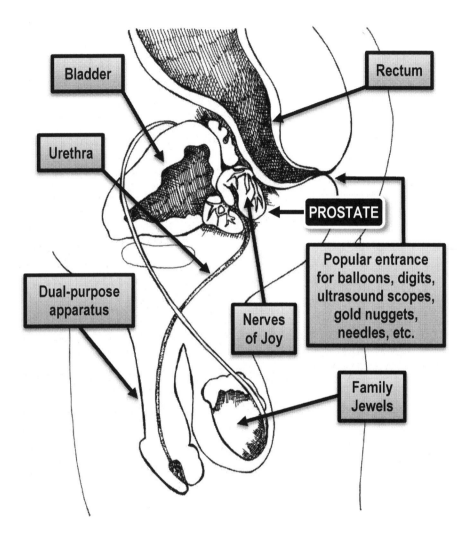

Bladder

Rectum

Urethra

PROSTATE

Popular entrance for balloons, digits, ultrasound scopes, gold nuggets, needles, etc.

Dual-purpose apparatus

Nerves of Joy

Family Jewels

It was unnerving that physicians and facilities offering any one of the treatment options were sure to claim theirs caused the least collateral damage, while enjoying cure rates equal to any. So I tried to always keep in mind that the world is not full of blatantly honest professionals eager to give totally frank and objective information to help me make an informed decision. Rather, the world is full of partially delusional, well-intentioned but misguided, highly biased, usually pleasant folks who have to ensure that the monthly payment for their gazillion dollar medical facility is made on time. To be fair, most of them probably do what they do well, but what they don't do is provide complete, unbiased information.

Except, of course, for my urologist, who is one of a rare breed. Email me and I'll send you his contact information.

After a week or so of stumbling around the Internet, researching on my own, I was ready to talk to someone who had been there and done that. With permission, Dr. Pee had given me the phone number of just such a guy—Harold—who had completed proton treatment in Florida in March 2010. I called him, we met at Barnes & Noble for coffee, and talked for several hours. Turns out he was a retired AP History teacher, and taught two of my four daughters in high school. Small world, but as I later learned, just about everybody has or will get prostate cancer. Except women (so far).

Harold was very upbeat, knowledgeable, candid, and positive about his choice to be treated at the University of Florida Proton Therapy Institute, and extremely pleased with the results. Minimal collateral damage. He pees a lot. Well, I already peed a lot before learning about my cancer. In fact, my wife pees now more than I did then, and only recently am I finally catching up with her. Our toilets are flushing all the time. More about peeing, later.

Harold was most encouraging, and then I was pleasantly and unexpectedly contacted by Bob[3], another former UFPTI proton patient. Bob saw my post on the Florida Proton online forum seeking advice about insurance issues. He noticed that we live not far from each other, was kind enough to contact me, offered to meet, and so I

---

[3] It turns out there are countless Bobs in the prostate cancer universe, and I have postulated that if your name is Bob you have a 33% greater chance of contracting prostate cancer. Sorry.

spent a few hours with him and his gracious wife in their home. He was also pleased with the results of his proton beam therapy, and thankful he found out about proton just a few days before his scheduled surgery, which he canceled.

It was becoming eerie. Both of these guys were happier than most people I know. Maybe even a little over the top. So I'm wondering, does proton treatment somehow make people happier? Is increased joyfulness a side effect of proton therapy? Or are these guys just nuts? I later learned that these guys are indeed nuts, but I genuinely like them, so I chose to believe them. And now I'm nuts, too. Be warned.

As my research continued, I discovered it is nearly impossible to find anything resembling an apples-to-apples study and comparison of prostate cancer treatment outcomes. This is partly because of the inherent competition between treatment modalities and facilities (e.g., *our protons are better than your protons*), and their understandable reluctance to share data with the competition. It is also due to the difficulty in measuring this at all. And finally, lots of guys treated for prostate cancer are (ahem) old, and die of something else before contributing much data to research. Personally, I intend to contribute a lot of data. As you know, I'm not old.

So it becomes necessary to find what you can, read what's available, add a few grains of salt to the whole mix, and glean an impression you can live with. And that's what I did. I gleaned.

The Decision Matrix

It's not really a matrix, but I like the way that sounds. Anyway, after about a month of research, I felt I had learned about all there was to find out. Here is a synopsis of my thinking:

I agreed with Dr. Pee that surgery was out. I wanted no knives anywhere near that stuff, especially the web of nerves around the prostate. Didn't want the urethra cut, either. I just don't much like the idea of all that cutting, although I know people who felt surgery was the only way to assuredly get rid of the cancer. On a visceral level, they wanted to just "get it out." I'm not one of those guys. To me, that was like throwing out the baby with the bath water.

And cryosurgery is, well, surgery. Freezing instead of cutting. Still sounds like hacking away at the prostate. Dr. Pee recommended against it, and he's my guy. Cryo was out.

At first I kind of liked the idea of brachytherapy, radioactive seeds implanted into the prostate, radiating from within. But I learned that the seeds can migrate to the lungs, the heart, and even under some circumstances (you can guess to which circumstances I refer), to my wife. This may or may not be troublesome; we just don't know yet. But to me, the "may" be troublesome part was troublesome. The notion of currently or formerly radioactive seeds forever having their way with me from the inside seemed, well, troublesome. Also, I don't like needles, and there are lots of needles involved in the seed implantation. Lots. And just to be sure, standard radiation is often combined with brachytherapy. Just to be sure? I don't like the way that sounds, either.

HIFU—high intensity focused ultrasound—might be interesting, and has a lot of characteristics that appealed to me. But it was not yet approved in the United States yet (still isn't), and I don't like to travel, even for something as fun as that sounds.

IMRT—intensity modulated radiation therapy—was closer to the mark. Blasting the prostate with radiation from the outside. No incisions, no cutting, no freezing, no needles, and painless. Sounds about right. Very high-tech. But here's the thing: the photon (X-ray) beam also radiates healthy tissue on the way to the prostate, and continues to radiate more healthy tissue on the other side, on the way out. So they have to change the angle a lot to try to minimize damage to the surrounding healthy tissue. You remember what healthy tissue I'm talking about: bladder, nerves, rectum, nerves. Remember that? The key word here is "try." The fact is, they can't help hitting the healthy tissue, both coming and going. They can only minimize the impact by moving the beam around. Still, it's the best sounding option so far.

But then, what does PBT—proton beam therapy—have to offer? It is also radiation, but shoots protons instead of the traditional photons as in IMRT. Well, very interesting. It turns out that protons have a unique characteristic, the Bragg Peak phenomenon, which places the bulk of the energy blast at the target (i.e., inside the prostate). Minimal intensity while entering, peak strength at the target, and near zero coming out the other side. I like the sound of this. Makes sense to me. Blast the diseased prostate from the outside, while barely touching the healthy stuff nearby.

Another proton factoid: it is almost impossible to find unhappy proton patients. Unlike patients of other approaches, proton guys seem almost universally happy with the results. Try to find some unhappy proton guys. You will have little success, if any.

And perhaps the most important, yet easily overlooked fact: "proton" spelled backwards, is:

NOTORP, or **No to R.P.**

R.P., of course, stands for radical prostatectomy. So proton itself cleverly embodies the rejection of the quite radical option of a prostatectomy, complete removal of the prostate. This little cited critical piece of data is what gave me the final push toward proton. So, so, clever, those proton people. The IMRT photon folks completely missed the boat on this. "Photon" spelled backwards is simply "No to H.P" and HP, as we all know, stands for Hewlett Packard. This is obvious irrelevant nonsense, and the IMRT photon crowd should be ashamed.

And if that isn't enough, read it forward: **pro**ton, and **pro**state. Duh! Clearly related terms with the same Latin derivation (I won't digress into a Latin lesson here). Now look at **pho**ton. What does that relate to? **Pho**tography? **Pho**tosynthesis? In fact, if you look up "pho" you'll find it's a Vietnamese noodle soup, not a cancer treatment.

Proton is indeed looking highly desirable, but what's its downside? Some say it's experimental, but it's not. They've been doing it for many years—even decades, depending upon how you measure—and expensive new facilities are cropping up all over the country and the world. If this is an experiment, it has become a monumentally huge one. The experiment is over. It works, but if you're uncomfortable with it, fine. Just don't do it. You don't need to fall back on the "experimental" rationalization to justify following a different route.

An often raised objection to proton treatment, and sometimes a show-stopper, is that it takes much longer than the alternatives. This is a valid issue. Currently, you'll need 6–8 weeks for proton, which can be inconvenient, difficult, unpleasant, and maybe even a little frightening for some guys, including me. I'm a homebody, and did not relish the idea of being even five hours away from home for so long. I like home. I don't like to travel. I don't even like long drives. I'm not especially fond of walking from one end of my house to the other. I like to stay put. It's been decades since I've been away from home for such an extended period. But I had to look at the big picture: Could I survive a couple months away from home for the best shot at a healthy rest-of-my-life? What am I, some kind of a wuss? Other guys, some possibly lesser than me, have survived the regimen. So can I. My son-in-law is currently somewhere on the other side of the globe on a naval aircraft carrier for six months or more. How bad can a couple months in Florida be?

I also didn't much like the idea of being away from my wife for so long. Wives often can and do accompany their husbands, but Lucy and I both work full time jobs, and she would not be able to take two months off to hold my hand in Florida. But she's more than a wife; she's also my best friend, and although nearly everyone treated at Florida Proton claims new friends-for-life will be made while there, I had my doubts about whether that would apply to me. I am very much a loner—even reclusive—and the idea that other guys would choose to befriend me seemed a little farfetched. I don't even play golf. So it looked like a lonely couple months, but again, in the overall context of life, I felt I could manage it if it meant staying out of diapers.

There is another time-related concern for those of us who are not yet retired: it could be difficult or impossible to miss up to eight weeks of consecutive work time. Fortunately, my employment situation was such that I was permitted and could afford to be away from full-time work for an extended period, and I am most appreciative of my employer for providing that flexibility. For some, this could be a show-stopper, but I was lucky to have the full support of my boss and organization. I was also able to work several hours via remote connection each day, which helped me remain sane and prevented me from falling too far behind with my work responsibilities.

All things considered, proton was the answer I was looking for, and I was ready and even eager to forge ahead. But there is one more downside to proton. A really big one. It is by far the most expensive option. So I now had to consider a potentially even harder question. Could I afford it?

Which leads me to the next chapter.

Your Money or Your Life

I had made my decision to aggressively pursue proton radiation therapy, but there were two more hurdles. Would the University of Florida Proton Therapy Institute accept me as a patient, and would my insurance company cover the treatment there? At my early stage of cancer (Gleason=3+3, Stage=t2a, PSA=5.9) I had no reason to fear Florida Proton would not want me. But the insurance decision-making process for something of this magnitude was a mystery to me, and I wasn't at all confident I'd be covered.

I contacted Florida Proton and received an overnight FedEx package the next day, which included a free copy of Bob Marckini's book. Did I mention that it's excellent, especially if you want useful, well-researched information? Along with the book you are now reading, what more do you need?

The cost of proton therapy can be a show stopper. The MSRP (manufacturer's suggested retail price) for the full Monty of protons is about $160,000. But don't worry, lunch is included every Wednesday for free. If you are personally footing the entire bill because you have no insurance coverage, a 15% discount (not quite, but almost as sweet as 20% off one item at Bed, Bath, and Beyond) was and might still be available, bringing the cost down to only $136,000. We are talking about some real savings here. I shopped at Publix yesterday and bought ten boxes of my favorite cereal on sale, two for $5. At first glance, you might think I was duped into spending a lot of money on cereal, but as it turns out I made about $20, no kidding! With proton treatment, you could pocket a whopping $24,000 in a hurry. Now that's what I'm talking about! This makes it worth considering proton therapy even if you don't have cancer or insurance.

And did I mention the free lunch?

Some insurance companies will not cover proton therapy, period. Others will consider it if it is deemed "medically necessary." Medically necessary? Really? Why do they think we want to do this? Just in case? Hardly necessary? A common refrain from these guys is that if you want to go with radiation, IMRT (the other radiation) is just as effective, but cheaper. It's a lucky thing Wal-Mart doesn't offer a treatment for prostate cancer (yet). If the only objective is to stop the cancer by any means—the cheaper, the better—without regard to future quality of life, why not just shoot me in the head? That'll stop the cancer, and a bullet is really cheap!

After researching the insurance issue, reading my policy, which also referred to the "medically necessary" issue without providing a clear, objective definition, and after talking with the helpful insurance staff at UFPTI, I was worried. In fact, I was much more concerned about financing the treatment than curing the cancer. Lucy and I began taking a personal inventory of what we'd have to sell to pay for proton without insurance, and the answer for us was simple: everything. So then we discussed whether it would be worth it. I mean, we love our home, but would we love it as much if I were in diapers, not peeing well, not pooping well, and unable to enjoy at least a brief roll in the hay on most Wednesday nights? Maybe a cheap efficiency apartment wouldn't be so bad.

My plan was to be aggressive about insurance, even if multiple appeals were needed, but I wanted to make my first pitch an effective one. Intuitively, I suspected that inclusion of a strongly worded referral letter from Dr. Pee would help. It would be great if he could ethically declare absolute indisputable medical necessity, but I doubted he'd be comfortable with that. However, he did write an excellent letter that came about as close as possible to claiming medical necessity without explicitly doing so. I could not have been happier or more appreciative.

In the meantime, in anticipation of the possible need to appeal I began building a list of others in my state of South Carolina who were insured by the same company, and were approved for proton treatment. This was not an easy task, as there is no handy list. I joined the UFPROTON user forum and found some help there, but my list was small.

Regardless, armed with a very strong referral letter from Dr. Pee, I sent my application to the University of Florida Proton Therapy Institute in Jacksonville, Florida, and they sent my application to the insurance company. I was lucky. My insurance company agreed to this therapy on the first try. No need to appeal. No need to sell the house. Or the kids.

YIPPEE! Research done, decision made, application accepted, insurance approved. DONE!

And that concludes the most technical couple of chapters in this book. Now, be honest, are you not totally impressed with my clear thinking, well-informed, impeccable reasoning? But remember, this was *my* thought process. You are entitled to your own. Whatever you do, *you* have to live with the consequences, as do I, as do we all. Just another HUGE decision that can't be avoided in this most interesting life.

You can agree with me or you can be wrong. The choice is yours.

Or you can do what Dr. Pee hinted at earlier. You can throw a dart to pick a treatment, but I'm not really a dart-throwing kind of guy. For me it was full steam ahead to proton, no looking back.

Instructions from Florida Proton

I soon received a nice little (by little, I mean big) packet of information from UFPTI—University of Florida Proton Therapy Institute—to help me prepare for the upcoming visit. Schedules, dietary restrictions, phone numbers of key personnel, and of course, the first of many, many forms to complete were included in this package. Thankfully, most of the forms could be completed online at my leisure, in advance of going to Jacksonville. I liked that a lot. It indicated that these folks have heard about technology and use it. It made me optimistic this also applied to the treatment I would receive at their facility. Real proton beam radiation—cool! Now, if only they could beam me over to Florida in a Star Trek style transporter, I'd be ecstatic.

Back to the forms: A number of them were questionnaires designed to track my side effect profile, my quality of life. These were lots of fun to fill out, and will voluntarily be filled out again and again periodically for the rest of my hopefully long life. How often do you have the opportunity to share with others your quality of peeing, pooping, and poking? By the way, I have observed that I and most of the guys I met during treatment lost all humility about these topics. They become every day, common fodder for chit chat. Barely even noteworthy. Coffee shop small talk.

Here's one survey question I found particularly memorable and amusing:

> *If you were to spend the rest of your life with*
> *your urinary symptoms just as they are now,*
> *how would you feel about that?*

The multiple-choice answers were: terrible, unhappy, mostly dissatisfied, equally satisfied & dissatisfied, mostly satisfied, pleased, or delighted. Delighted? Really? Is that a sentiment anyone would typically consider using to describe urinary performance?

You: Hey, Ron, how's it going?

Me: Great, thanks, and may I say that today I'm just delighted with my urinary performance? Really. Just delighted! It's a fine day, and if you'll excuse me, I'm going to enjoy another wonderfully delightful pee right now. Back in a jiffy!

On another questionnaire, the one about sexual function, I especially enjoyed this insightful, probing question:

On average, how often do you have sexual intercourse or achieve erections suitable for it?

This is a very dignified way of asking for your batting average. Five possible answers were provided: never, once a month, twice a month, once a week, or twice a week. I'm not sure how you would answer if your average were, say, three, four, or five times a week. Maybe there's a different questionnaire for such superstars. If I were a five times a week guy, I'd feel really cheated to have to answer twice a week, that being the closest available answer, and there is no provision to answer in essay format or add explanatory comments. If you were a 5x guy forced to answer 2x, wouldn't you feel robbed? I suppose the questionnaire gurus had a meeting, identified the demographic, and decided that hey, what are the chances any of these guys can make it happen more than twice a week? Hahaha! Zip. Zero. Nada. No need to include a "two or more times a week" option. Can't happen. Not with this bunch of geezers.

Regardless of the question committee's misconceptions about us, we in this demographic like to be accurate, we like to be honest, and we like to be correctly represented in important matters. The restrictive and limited choice of answers makes this difficult if not impossible, and we would very possibly be forced to round our answers to the closest available option. But alas, there were no instructions about how to deal with rounding, a glaring oversight by the quiz gods.

For example, if the answer is sometimes once a week, sometimes twice a week, then which do you choose to be honest and accurate? The answer is 1.5 times, on average. I am guessing most of us would round up, as a small and harmless ego boost. This will skew the results because those in the twice weekly, more than twice weekly, and 1½ times weekly groups would all have to choose the twice weekly option, making it a larger group than it really is. Those interpreting the survey would be misled into thinking that "two" is the magic number for proton guys. Maybe it is, maybe it isn't.

Things become totally ridiculous when you consider the second half of the question, the "or achieve erections suitable for it" part. That can *really* make the survey misleading, at best. This part of the question is only a thinly disguised way of asking how often we *could* do it, if given the opportunity. Let's see now, there was a pretty good opportunity at 3am, but I didn't want to wake Lucy, but that still counts. Then woops—again when my alarm clock rang, so that's two. Add to those a possible actual encounter with Lucy's participation and my score is already three for that day, which could become twenty-one times *on average* for the week if I keep up the same pace. Why, I do believe I am some kind of a superhero!

So when you consider both halves of the question, it turns out that the first part, "How often do you have sexual intercourse," is irrelevant. Taken in its entirety, this question could be stated more concisely and directly:

How often could you do it if you wanted to?

The two sample questions above are representative of many others, so be prepared and forewarned: there will be lots of probing questions about topics you probably never expected to be discussing much, especially because many of us are from a generation where discussion of such issues was usually confined to the locker room, where we mostly lied to each other. But answer the questions, and be truthful. It's important for creating meaningful statistical data about side effect profiles of prostate treatment, and future prostate cancer victims will appreciate your effort.

Filling out the forms was fun, but not as challenging as figuring out what I was allowed to eat. The UFPTI package contained several pages of dietary rules and guidelines, which boiled down to just two words: don't eat. Anything that could cause any digestive distress whatsoever, especially gaseousness (i.e., farting), was absolutely off the menu. In my case, that would rule out everything edible. So I voluntarily gave up beans, pretty much ignored the rest of the eating doctrine, and kept my fingers crossed that no one would notice my lack of diligence. However, Lucy did notice the positive effect of eliminating beans and was openly pleased with the result. She encouraged me to give them up for good, as it was a positive step for the "green" movement, resulting in a more habitable atmosphere for the entire planet.

I still eat beans.

Get Ready, Get Set

It was November 2010, about a month after I was diagnosed. I was shifting into high gear now. All signals were go, and there was a lot to do. First on the agenda: as part of my pre-qualification for treatment, Florida Proton needed a recent colonoscopy. When I called Dr. Gastro (a clever pseudonym for my gastroenterologist) who years ago did a spectacular job (translation: I remember nothing about it), I learned that December is the busy season for colonoscopies and he was booked solid. Who would have guessed that long tubes up your butt was a seasonal thing? Do people give colonoscopy gift cards as Christmas presents? No, the reason for the December butt rush is insurance-related, as is much of life. Colonoscopants (I made that word up, so don't add it to your spell-checker) want to get it done within the current calendar year, before their insurance deductible resets on the first of January.

Good point. In fact, my oldest daughter Julie had previously advised me to try, if possible, to do as much as I could within a single calendar year to minimize my out of pocket costs. I have smart kids, protecting their inheritance at every opportunity. So I begged and pleaded with Dr. Gastro, played the cancer card for sympathy, and he (or to be fair, it was his nurse) agreed to work me in on December 3rd. Perfect. I could hardly wait. That would hopefully allow me time to also complete the pre-treatment requirements at Florida Proton within the same calendar year, with actual treatments beginning in January. From an insurance standpoint, this would work well. Here's why, and it's kind of interesting:

Phase 1 includes the initial consultation with your oncologist, plus a CT scan of the pelvic area. Phase 2 includes a bone scan, chest X-ray, MRI, fiducial marker implantation, and finally the simulation (involving another CT scan, an open MRI, and fabrication of my body pod). I'll describe these in detail later, but the point now is that these are costly procedures done at both the University of Florida Proton Therapy Institute and the neighboring Shands Hospital facilities. These tests are followed by a plethora of big bills trickling in for several months from everyone you've seen and everywhere you've been, representing potentially the biggest out-of-pocket chunk of the whole proton deal. So as Julie said, it is important for all of the above to occur in the same calendar year.

In contrast, Phase 3, the treatment phase, is billed to the patient at the copay cost for an office visit to a specialist. In my case, this was $35 per visit, and was not subject to any deductible, so it didn't matter if it was in the same calendar year as the other procedures. It would add up to an estimated $1,750 for my 39 treatments and a few additional visits, regardless of when they occurred. So from an insurance standpoint, the key was to complete the colonoscopy, Phase 1, and Phase 2 in the same calendar year. I just barely made it, finishing them all before the end of 2010, but in this case, close enough is good enough.

With a commitment for an updated colonoscopy, as well as a copy of my most recent lab work (PSA, etc.) Florida Proton was willing to schedule me for Phase 1 (the 1-day consultation) and Phase 2 (the 3-day workup and simulation). These are usually done on separate visits, the idea being that after the consultation either they or I might decide to shake hands and go our separate ways, no hard feelings. However, as stated, I was in high gear and there was a near zero chance I'd change my mind, so I asked and Florida agreed to schedule a combined Phase 1 + Phase 2 visit, which they are willing to consider when the likelihood of not proceeding is low. The combined visit would typically occur on four consecutive days, Monday through Thursday, or Tuesday through Friday, but because this was right before Christmas, my Phase 1 consultation was set for Friday, December 17, followed by the Phase 2 jamboree starting on Monday, December 20. That gave us a weekend to enjoy Jacksonville between phases.

So the colonoscopy was scheduled, Phases 1 and 2 were set, and now we (Lucy could thankfully accompany me on this trip) needed to find a place to stay in Jacksonville. The local guys (Harold and Bob) with whom I spoke earlier had their favorite spots, and the Florida Proton website has a wealth of excellent information on their website, www.floridaproton.org. If proton therapy ever falls out of favor, they could easily morph into a travel agency instead. Where you stay is entirely a matter of personal preference, of course. You can choose to be close to the treatment facility, near the beaches, south of the St. Johns River, or in the area north of the facility. All are described conveniently on the website.

We chose to make reservations at a relatively new gated apartment complex primarily for UFPTI patients, family, and friends called Third and Main, an easy five minute drive from the facility. They had the right combination of amenities for me, and this is where I stayed for all three phases. They were about as nearby as possible to the place I'd have to visit every weekday, and even with my Garmin, I'm not good at and don't like driving around unfamiliar towns. That's just me, though. You might not care.

Also being and knowing me, I knew that without an on-premises exercise room, I would not exercise. The YMCA offers a special rate for Florida Proton patients, but that was irrelevant to me. I wouldn't go, and I knew it. Third and Main has a small exercise room with a treadmill, elliptical, bike, and weights, and this ultimately worked out well for me. My abs of steel and envious physique were maintained. Just ask anyone, or look at the book cover and let your imagination run wild.

There are a couple deli-type restaurants on the ground floor below the Third and Main apartments on the second and third floors. Very convenient, indeed. And just a few blocks down Main Street were a little Greek restaurant, a Chinese drive-through, a post office, a branch of my bank, and just across the street, a little quick-stop gas station. What more could I need, aside from a healthier prostate?

My colonoscopy was set, my labs were scheduled, our reservation at Third and Main was confirmed, and my Phase 1 / Phase 2 workup appointments were on the books. Now it was just a short wait until hitting the road for Jacksonville.

Go! Florida Phase 1

On Thursday, December 16th, 2010, Lucy and I were on the road to Florida in my snazzy 2007 Chrysler Pacifica (a crossover vehicle, <u>not</u> a minivan, which would be totally uncool) by 4:30. It's a straight shot, I-26 south to I-95, then south into Jacksonville. As easy as that would be for most people, I was not only a cancer victim, but also seriously direction-disabled, relying entirely on my Garmin and Lucy to keep

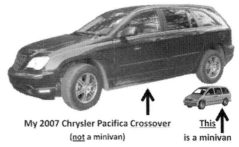

My 2007 Chrysler Pacifica Crossover (<u>not</u> a minivan)   This ↑ is a minivan

me moving south. Thankfully, one of my two afflictions has now been remedied, but the other seems to be incurable (proton can't fix everything). We stopped once for a quick dinner and arrived at Third and Main at about 10:00 to quickly unpack and go to bed (in the sleep sort of way). This was to be my home for two full months in January, so I had my fingers crossed that this preview of coming accommodations would work out well, and it did.

I was apprehensive. Lots to worry about. Both Harold and Bob described the 3-day workup as the worst part of the entire experience, involving busy schedules and a long line of guys and gals wanting to poke, prod, and otherwise invade my personal space. And right from the start, the looming MRI had me especially worried. I am claustrophobic and had no interest in being loaded into the infamous, ominous MRI tube. I was not looking forward to any of this, but at least I knew it would be over one way or the other by Wednesday. Also, Lucy's accompaniment on this trip was extremely comforting, and as it turned out, quite useful.

Friday morning we were up at six and had a good (by good, I mean big) breakfast downstairs at Uptown Market. Crisp, thick, applewood smoked bacon and … who can remember, and what does it matter? Crisp, thick applewood smoked bacon says it all.

I was scheduled to be at the University of Florida Proton Therapy Institute at 8:30, and was directed to start fasting at 8:00 to prepare for my upcoming CT scan. It was literally a five minute drive from Third and Main, and there is a patient-only gated parking lot just a few steps from the front door of the building. I had been given the code, and I still have the code. I will love, cherish, and protect the code, as I'm not often entrusted with secret codes for much of anything. If you want to know the code, I'm sorry. I can't help you. You must get cancer to find out the code. If I find myself anywhere in Jacksonville I will certainly go there, just so I can use the code again. I love codes. But I will not tell you the code. If I did, I'd have to kill you.

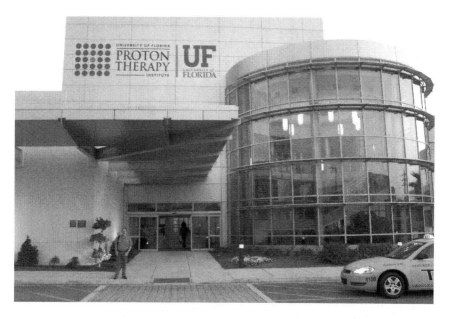

The Florida Proton building is modern, bright, spacious, and well-appointed. The main waiting area is more like the lobby of an above average hotel. There are comfortable easy chairs, a baby grand piano, water cooler, coffee bar, small library, jigsaw puzzle table, and even a children's game room. A PowerPoint slide show on a monitor above the coffee bar continually announces patient information and social events, and a smiling concierge at a semi-circular desk greets you as soon as you enter the building. By concierge I mean young, attractive, friendly, competent female receptionist. My understanding is that most of the prostate cancer patients are guys, so this was a nice touch, and as turned out, a preview of coming attractions.

Notably absent in the lobby was a TV. This omission was apparently intended to promote social interaction between the patients. How silly! What better way could there be to interact than to watch CNN or Fox News together? Oh, well. Patients and families were given no choice, and seemed willing enough to talk with each other.

But this morning we spent no time in the lobby. Our first Phase 1 visit was at 8:30 with UFPTI's financial counselor. This involved signing a stack of agreements and forking over the estimated $1,750 of anticipated copays for the Phase 3 treatments. I reminded myself that Wednesday lunches would be free, and happily handed over the loot.

Next stop: meet my case manager—let's call her Casey—so designated by virtue of being Dr. Candor's (not his real name) nurse. By the way, I forgot to mention that Dr. Candor is the newest member of my crack[4] medical team, and my designated UFPTI oncologist. Dr. Candor is laid back, and (big surprise) a first-rate shrugger, having refined it to an artful degree of subtlety and natural delivery even Dr. Perry and Dr. Pee would admire.

Casey had (surprise again) a stack of paperwork needing my signature, and as a bonus, a couple jugs of barium solution for me to drink in preparation for the CT scan two hours later. She claimed that some people say the solution tastes like a piña colada minus the

---

[4] I have been informed by two of my daughters (Jessica and Emily, both well-educated) that they are unfamiliar with this use of the word *crack*, so I must assume there might be other readers confused as well. I am using definition #44 from dictionary.com, which defines *crack* as *first-rate; excellent: a crack shot.* Later in this book I use the term *crackerjack*, which urbandictionary.com defines as *excellent; outstanding in quality or ability.* They label this usage as *dated* and *informal.* Well, maybe so. I still like it.

I most vividly remember Johnny Carson's frequent use of *crack* in his opening monologues on the Tonight Show, in which he sarcastically referred to *NBC's crack meteorologist* as the butt of many weather-related jokes. They made me laugh, and I like the word.

If you're not sure whether you belong to my generation or that of Jessica and Emily, you can use your understanding of *crack* as a litmus test. As a follow-up test, ask yourself who was the best host ever of The Tonight Show. Nope, not Jack Paar or Steve Allen. Not Leno. Conan who?

liquor. I beg to differ. To me it tasted like a barium solution. Maybe a fancy glass and a tiny umbrella would have helped dupe me.

Next, meet Dr. Candor, who nobly met with me as scheduled despite an obvious serious cold. Dr. Candor is personable, has a pleasant bedside manner, is old enough to have considerable experience, but young enough to still be interested and actively engaged in his field. As it turned out, this meeting was my longest with Dr. Candor. It was the official Phase 1 consultation, part of the screening process to see if UFPTI and I met each other's criteria to proceed with treatment. I was on my best behavior, which is unfortunately not so good.

Naturally, I needed to know whether Dr. Candor could administer an effective DRE, and I insisted he do so before I would agree to any further discussion. Oh, wait; maybe it was the other way around. Anyway, as mentioned earlier, Dr. Candor's technique, which took me by surprise, involved me on my back, legs apart, knees up. This approach, he explained, just happens to be the way he was taught to do it. And a fine job he does, indeed. Quick and easy, without fanfare. He was satisfied with what he found (or what he failed to find), and I was satisfied, too. Everyone was happy, but only I had cancer and no one else would join me in a barium toast.

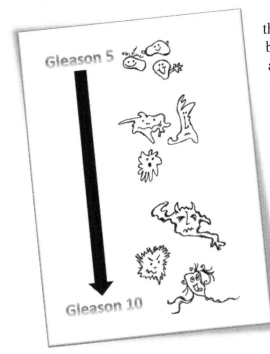

Dr. Candor confirmed that my biopsy slides had been reevaluated, and it was agreed that my Gleason score was 6, as originally stated. This relieved one of my lingering concerns, that my Gleason might be deemed higher than the original score of 6. This score is extremely important, as it is the primary measurement of the aggressiveness of the cancer cells. Higher scores indicate meaner cells, lower scores mean happy face cells.

It was Dr. Pee who explained this to me the prior month back home in South Carolina when he first broke the big "C" news to me. Dr. Pee took a scrap of paper and sketched little circles of happy faces, not-so-happy slightly mutated faces, and finally, unmistakably mean, unhappy grotesquely distorted faces. These artful little dudes represented cancer cells at various Gleason scores. It would take a score of 5 or less to see lots of happy faces, which would be unusual. My score was 6. Not so happy, but not real mean, either. That's good news for me. Scores in the 7–9 range would be troublesome, indicating more aggressive cancer cells.

So why did UFPTI have to agree that my score was 6 when it had already been determined to be 6, you might ask, as did I. It turns out that characterizing the little happy-mean faces of the cancer cells is highly subjective. One person might see somber faces, while another sees those same faces as agitated little fellows, depending on what everybody had for breakfast. I know someone whose biopsy slides were initially labeled as Gleason 6, then upped to Gleason 7 upon reevaluation, and finally declared a Gleason 8 from a hopefully tie-breaking third opinion that only made matters more confusing. Two more opinions and he might have become a perfect 10. Same slides, three different interpreters, three different scores. Dr. Candor's agreement that I was indeed a 6 meant I'd need no additional opinions, and I was probably a solid 6. Two for two. If you ever hoped for a perfect 10, this was not the time. I was a solid 6, and glad of it.

With a Gleason 6, and without much prostate enlargement or palpable (meaning detectable via the finger up the butt) tumor, I was well on my way to approval for proton therapy. Dr. Candor then launched into an extremely thorough, informative, and well-practiced description of the history of developments in the treatment of prostate cancer, including mention of his prior experience specializing in brachytherapy—radioactive seed implants. He explained that during the period when he was involved with seeds, brachytherapy was cutting edge treatment, but now proton radiation had advantages and was by far the best option for me at my early stage.

The usual treatment package involved 39 daily (Monday through Friday) proton zaps, which is what I was prepared for. However, there is also a newer 28 day plan that results in the same cumulative amount of radiation in bigger spoonfuls each time. Cutting two weeks off my Florida trip was certainly appealing, but alas, I did not qualify. I have an internal hemorrhoid, knocking me out of the running for the short course. Darn that hemorrhoid. It was proving to be a menace in more ways than one. So, despite some feeble pleading, I would need all 39 proton blasts.

The next part of Dr. Candor's presentation caught me off guard, and was contrary to what my research indicated. He was crystal clear that after proton therapy, my pecker would not be doing much poking. This condition is commonly referred to as "ED," first discovered in the late 1990s by Bob Dole (shortly before Al Gore invented the Internet). I knew ED—erectile dysfunction—was a possibility, along with incontinence, but my impression was that the likelihood of either was perhaps lower (again, no unequivocal apples-to-apples comparative studies) with proton than other approaches. At least that was what I surmised from my conversations and research.

Now, while we guys certainly don't want either incontinence or erectile dysfunction, the latter is usually the less troublesome of the two. Incontinence could be a 24/7/365 problem, while ED would only be a problem Wednesday nights. All things considered, if a choice must be made, ED is the logical choice. But I was not of the impression that it was a forgone conclusion, which is essentially how Dr. Candor presented it. That is also how the medical release form presented it. Despite this, I continued to believe proton offered the best chance of avoiding both incontinence and ED, so I signed the papers. And I can thankfully report that right now, as my beloved late mother-in-law once cleverly wrote as a festive message on a birthday cake she baked and decorated for my wife's 42nd birthday, it's "so far, so good." And I know many other guys who are still enjoying Wednesday nights, so I must assume Dr. Candor was bound to present a worst-case-scenario as a CYA for UFPTI, and that's understandable. I think it amounted to an "expect the worst, hope for the best" approach. Nevertheless, I was not in the frame of mind to expect the worst. I was counting on the best, and counting on protons to deliver for me. So far, so good.

Toward the end of our meeting with Dr. Candor, he wrote a bunch of prescriptions, most notably for some antibiotics to start taking two days before the gold marker procedure, to prevent infection. But I needed one more prescription, and did not hesitate to ask for it. Nor did he hesitate to provide it. I knew I would need a little help with the MRI tube, and he was happy to prescribe a Valium-like sedative. This prescription is not a standard part of the goody bag, and I'm glad I thought to ask for it. I'm sure the MRI technicians are also glad.

Before we finished, Dr. Candor had one more delightful tidbit of news for me.

The Infamous Balloon

Dr. Candor explained that one of the objectives during radiation of the prostate is to minimize the amount of surface area it shares with the rectal wall. Marckini described how a specialized balloon is used for that purpose at Loma Linda. In fact, Bob's website (www.protonbob.org) and his organization use the acronym BOB: Brotherhood of the Balloon. And Marckini's first name is Bob, too. It was clearly his destiny.

Here's how it works: An empty balloon is delicately slipped into the rectum and then filled with a saline solution to inflate it. Most radiation therapists understandably prefer this inflation method to blowing it up in the usual way, and this has become the standard operating procedure. Once inflated, the balloon pulls the rectum away from the prostate, and the rectal wall then receives relatively little of the radiation aimed at the prostate. Clever little system, I must admit. This was a medically sound solution to a challenging problem, while also being an ingenious public relations technique promoting proton therapy to the countless guys like myself who have always had a happy, festive feeling about balloons. I mean, who doesn't love balloons, right?

Before I knew the above details of the balloon technique, I was vaguely aware of it and had therefore asked Harold and Bob about it. But they each told me Florida Proton no longer used the balloon, so any balloon talk was purely academic and would not apply to me, which initially was a relief. As much as I do like balloons, there is a time and a place, and, well, that might have been the right time, but surely seemed like the wrong place.

But not to worry, said Harold and Bob. There'd be no balloons for me. In Florida, instead of the balloon they shoot saline straight up the butt without a balloon. Doesn't that sound lovely? I recall being more than a little distressed and concerned about that approach, and simply could not imagine how it would work in practice. I'm supposed to do what? Squeeze my butt cheeks as if trying not to poop (I guess) for how long? It's totally up to me to keep the juice in its place until they finish with the beam? I had serious doubts I could pull that off, and both guys did mention that as soon as their treatment was over they made a mad dash to the nearby restroom to let the liquid loose. I spent the better part of a month trying to wrap my brain around how to accomplish this unnatural feat, and could not quite get there.

But surprise, surprise! Dr. Candor explained that Florida Proton determined that although the saline approach worked well in most cases, the balloon was more consistent. Therefore, they had returned to using the balloon exclusively, and I would soon become a balloon boy after all. This was ... great news. As I said, I love balloons. However, the idea of a balloon up my butt was admittedly a new concept and would take some adjustment in my thinking and expectations[5]. Especially an estimated total of 40 balloons (not at the same time).

I hoped each would be a different, festive color.

_____

[5] I have included a detailed description of the actual balloon experience in the Phase 2: Simulation chapter, and also in the Phase 3: Treatments chapter.

Phase 1: My First Tube

I was now finished with Dr. Candor, and Lucy and I left the Florida Proton building with instructions for the remainder of the day. CT scan day. This would be our first encounter with the Shands medical facilities, where most of the imaging is done. They are not part of UFPTI, or vice versa, and the atmosphere is more clinical. The small, unassuming one-level building for the CT scan was just down the street from the Florida Proton Institute. Inside, the patient waiting area sported rows of typical waiting room chairs, random magazines, and very busy personnel doing their best not to fall behind schedule as they gathered the required data, forms, and signatures from the UFPTI referrals and other patients.

Although we had an appointment, we had to wait for about two hours, sufficient time to allow my frazzling nerves to frazzle even more. But my state of mind began to improve once it was finally my turn to enter Shands' inner sanctum. There, the very nice people involved in performing the scan were professional and caring, could sense my apprehension, and were surprisingly successful in addressing and relieving much of my anxiety. And anxious I was: this was not the MRI tube, but it was a tube nonetheless. More like a donut, into which I would slide on a table feet first, with my head never entering. I was happy to learn my head would be spared (this was a scan of the pelvic area). I'm not sure why, but I prefer keeping my head outside of tubes, donuts, or whatever, and that gave me some small comfort.

Next, they inserted an IV needle into my right arm for the purpose of injecting an iodine solution for imaging contrast. That iodine is some weird stuff, and had the IV injector person not described its effect to me in advance, I would have undoubtedly panicked. But thankfully, she explained I would experience an immediate, strong metallic taste, followed by internal warmth that would rapidly spread from my head to my buttocks, and then stop. She was spot on right. It was intense, and I'm sure glad she forewarned me or I would have thought it was curtains. In hindsight, it was pretty cool. A drug producing that kind of sensation would have a hefty black market price. You could start to like it, especially if it could be made to last. But I was not in the right frame of mind and failed to appreciate the iodine rush at the time. Oh, well. So in went the iodine, and in went me. I kept my eyes closed, which helped, and the scan itself was relatively quick, lasting just a few minutes. In, out, done. Really, no big deal. What a baby am I.

And that, my friends, concludes Phase 1 of the Florida Proton experience. Well, sort of. Lucy and I now had our first opportunity for a relaxed meal and went to Town Center Mall, a huge outdoor complex of stores and restaurants they refer to as a mall. Back home a mall is a small indoor building shared by some stores and a food court. We had a tasty lunch at California Pizza, sitting outside, glad that weather permitted. Then I began a rapid descent into fatigue, we went back to the apartment, and I had diarrhea for the rest of the day. I am guessing it was a reaction to the iodine, barium, or both. Odd. I don't usually react that way to barium and iodine, do you?

While I was occupied with the above, Lucy went out to do a little grocery shopping and fill the prescriptions for medication I would need to start taking on Sunday. We had popcorn, watched the last two episodes of In Treatment Season 2, and went to bed.

Saturday was much better. No lingering effects from the iodine or barium. Just to be safe, I had nothing more than an English muffin for breakfast. There would be plenty of time for more bacon later. That afternoon we rendezvoused with my brother-in-law Scott who made the drive from Gainesville to see us. It was another beautiful day, and we met at San Marco Square, walked around a while, lunched at the San Marco Deli, and then adjourned to Starbucks to extend our visit. It's amazing how much time you can kill at Starbucks. Afterward, Lucy and I had dinner at San Marco Pizza and returned to the apartment. All in all, this was a pleasant, relaxing day, with none of the ill effects of the day before.

On Sunday I filled my belly with another (ahem) modest little breakfast at Uptown Market. Then we went to The Avenues Mall, had a surprisingly excellent lunch later at Bob Evans, shopped around here and there, exploring Jacksonville in a random way, returned to the apartment, nuked a couple of Lean Cuisines (our standard dinner fare back home), watched TV, and went to bed. Notably, I also started antibiotics in preparation for the gold marker placement Tuesday. To prevent infection, you start those meds two days prior to, and continue until two days after that procedure.

The next morning, Monday, Phase 2 would begin. I was not looking forward to it. It was MRI day, and even with sedatives in hand, I was apprehensive. This was not the CT scan donut. This was the dreaded tube, head first, and tooooo small. I was counting on the magic pills to perform as expected.

Phase 2: Poking & Prodding

The big day arrived. MRI Monday. Hooray! And in case that wasn't exciting enough, there was more. It was bone scan day, too. And even that wasn't all. It was also chest X-ray day. Now tell me, could I possibly have asked for more?

I started the day at 10:00 again with Shands, but this time at a larger, more hospital-like facility than the cute little CT scan shack of the prior day. There I met with the technician who would administer a full body bone scan. I'll call him Bones (not his real name, and probably no relation to Star Trek's Dr. "Bones" McCoy). He needed to give me an injection a couple hours prior to the scan, but first I asked him how the bone scan was done, and guess what! Another freaking tube! I didn't much like the looks of it, either, and my reaction was not lost on Bones. He was savvy, and wisely invited me to check it out, climb aboard, and give it a quick spin to see if I was okay with it. If not, he correctly reasoned, there was no point wasting the injection on me. This was extremely kind and sensitive of Bones, wonderful customer service, and as it turned out, his tube was not bad at all. So I got the shot, and moved on to the next item on my agenda.

It was back to Florida Proton for more engrossing paperwork with Casey, my case manager. I don't know how much medical training she has, but she is certainly experienced with forms. We reviewed the schedule for the remainder of Phase 2, finished with her at about noon, went back to Uptown Market for lunch, and then had a few minutes to relax upstairs in our suite. We were clearly becoming regulars at Uptown, and why not? They offered a 10% discount for proton patients, no ID required. So even *you* could dine there and claim your discount if you are unscrupulous. Not too sure if it would work for a woman.

Then it was back to see Bones at Shands for the scan, which took about a half hour to gradually move me through the tube, feet first. Or maybe the tube moved over me. I can't really remember. Feeling quite proud to have notched another scan on my belt, we played our "get a chest X-ray whenever you find time" wild card, since we were already in the right place. We went upstairs, I got the required chest X-ray without any waiting, and crossed it off my list.

The fun part of the day was over. It was now back to the Shands Scan Shack for the dreaded MRI. I popped one of the Valium knockoffs about an hour beforehand, as directed. I felt nothing, and was sure this pill was a placebo. Shands was estimating a wait of an hour or two, so I panicked a little about whether and when to take another pill, and since it was unclear exactly how long it would be before they'd be ready for me, I had to guess. So placebo or not, I popped another pill just to be sure. Still felt nothing. Oh, no. It wasn't working. I was going to die of MRI shock.

Finally it was my turn. I instructed Lucy that if I didn't return in a reasonable amount of time she should storm the "authorized personnel only" door and rescue me. So in I went, and again, the technicians were friendly and most sensitive to my concerns. I got comfortable on the table, and into the tube of horrors I went, head first. In fact, my head went all the way through the tube, and when the table stopped moving I looked up to see daylight and the technician standing there reassuringly. She left me there, went into the control room, and a most entertaining cacophony of clanks, buzzes, and shakes began. It was somewhat hypnotic, and I found it easy to focus on those special effects. I mean, they could have just left me laying there in silence, but for me they went to the trouble of providing this amazing percussion concert.

Then it was done, and out I came. Not bad at all! It didn't matter that the meds did nothing; I amazingly almost enjoyed the experience, totally on my own. I rule. I am great. I can have an MRI and live to tell about it. I shared this revelation with Lucy, and she grinned, explaining that this was exactly what those little pills were supposed to accomplish, and how wonderful it was they worked so well for me. So it turns out I'm not so great after all, but so what. I was done with the tube FOREVER!

We are creatures of habit and went back to California Pizza for dinner, then to the apartment, chilled out in front of the TV, and went to bed. We did not go back for another MRI.

Tuesday, the second day of Phase 2, began with breakfast in the apartment, two pain pills, and a Fleets enema, which I administered myself. I can't exactly remember how I did it. I had never given myself an enema before and had to wing it. One way or another, this unnatural act had the desired result. Cleaned me out pretty well. I was proud of myself, and so was Lucy, who was spared the job of providing any assistance with this.

The pain pills and enema were in preparation for the next procedure on the hit parade of poking and prodding: the insertion of four gold markers, known as fiducial markers, into my prostate. Yes, I would have seeds implanted after all. However, these little guys were just your ordinary, everyday seeds, not the fancy radioactive ones used in brachytherapy. Just four little gold nuggets the size of a grain of wild rice. Yum.

We arrived at 9:30 in the urologist's office (holy smokes, now I have TWO urologists) for the marker implantation. Of course, the seeds are implanted via the tunnel to paradise (my rectum), and those who had already had this done sometimes described it as a *biopsy lite*. As you'll recall, I was not present for my biopsy, so for me this was my first conscious procedure of scopes and needles up my butt to stick stuff into my prostate. One notable difference between this and a biopsy: this guy was only putting stuff in, not taking stuff out. I think that matters. What's mine is mine, after all. You can't just go up my butt and take what you want whenever you want to, you know.

Anyway, this procedure was done with local anesthetic, took about fifteen minutes, and was indeed relatively painless. Yes, there was some minor *discomfort* (ahem)—a few quick jabs of tolerable pain—but I preferred it to traveling through another tube. So I was now packing gold.

By the way, the purpose of the markers is for X-ray detection of the position of the prostate during treatments. The prostate moves around a little, so they have to determine precisely where it currently is each time they shoot the beam. The low-dose X-ray sees the markers, and the table is adjusted to align me and my prostate properly. Wouldn't want them to miss the mark, no sirree bob. BOB? Oops. More on BOB later.

I was feeling rather upbeat, seeing light at the end of the tunnel. Lucy and I lunched at a little home cooking dive of a restaurant where the meatloaf was rather tasty and the waitress was a super duper friendly ol' gal, mighty proud of their meatloaf. We then did a little more shopping around town, and returned to UFPTI for the facility tour, which was optional. I'm glad we did the tour, though. I was able to take a quick peek into a treatment room for the first time. Wow! This was impressive, and I'll describe it in detail later. On the tour, suffice it to say I was stunned and awed that I was going to visit one of the three rooms every weekday for two months. Stunned. Awed.

Then it was home for a marvelous Lean Cuisine dinner, a movie, and bed. Just one day to go!

I woke up Wednesday, the third and final day of Phase 2, not feeling too well. I felt weak, had a headache, and was a little nauseous. I chalked it up to the restriction of having no caffeine that morning. I am addicted to caffeine. I need my caffeine every morning. Lots of it, or I will surely have a headache soon enough. I need my coffee. With caffeine. Please.

Caffeine-deprived, off I went to the Institute where all of the remaining work was to be done by the happy, friendly folks at Florida Proton. I wonder if they had their caffeine. Probably. Couldn't be that happy otherwise.

Phase 2: Simulation

This third and final day of the workup phase is referred to as the simulation, a dry run for what would become my daily treatment regimen. There were some additional things that had to be done during simulation that would not be part of the daily routine, but overall, this was a rehearsal with everything but the proton beam. In fact, it was a dress rehearsal, in costume. I had studied my lines, and was as ready as I could be to play my part. I was in the starring role.

So, here we go. We arrived at the Institute, checked in at the desk, and found a couple of comfortable easy chairs. One of the smiling radiation therapists—not a clerk, and not a paper shuffler, but an actual therapist who administers treatments—personally greeted us and instructed me to empty my bladder (translation: pee it all out) and then drink the two glasses of water he brought me from the nearby cooler, about 15 ounces total. First you empty, and then you drink. This routine is cleverly referred to as "empty and drink." The objective is to put the bladder in a predictable, repeatable, filled condition. A full bladder is extremely important to protect the bladder from the proton beam. The bladder kind of drapes itself over the prostate, but when it's full it plumps up, pulling away from the prostate, minimizing the amount of surface contact with it. That way the beam touches very little of the bladder, and when the therapy is done my bladder should still work pretty well. Good plan.

A full bladder does for the bladder what the balloon does for the rectum. The objective is to isolate the prostate as much as possible, while simultaneously helping to stabilize its position during treatment. My feeling is that the balloon and "empty and drink" are also at least partly to make sure the entire treatment isn't too easy and therefore not at all memorable. The proton beam itself cannot be felt, but fortunately the balloon and full bladder are quite noticeable, and I cherish these memories.

RT#1 (radiation therapist #1) said he'd return to retrieve me in about 30 minutes, and indeed he did. He and the pretty RT#2 took me to the changing room where I was asked to replace my pants and underwear with a lovely white polka dotted gown, open at the back, and tied at the neck. I was allowed to keep my shirt and socks on, which left me feeling, well, half naked. I locked the rest of my clothes in the small locker and put the stylish elastic key bracelet around my wrist. Then I flung open the dressing room curtain, threw my arms up into the air, shouted "TA DA!" and waited for applause. Instead, I was politely escorted into the simulation room.

The objectives of simulation are to confirm the amount of water and length of time required to fill my bladder, to calibrate the balloon for the size and depth of my rectum, to confirm proper placement of the gold fiducial markers, to create my personal "pod" (explained below), and to obtain 3-D imagery needed to customize a brass aperture and Lucite lens to the exact shape of my prostate. All of this is to help ensure that the proton beam hits the target (and only the target) as precisely and thoroughly as possible. I'm for that, yes indeed.

I climbed up onto the table (referred to by some as the "slab"), as instructed. Actually, I climbed onto a flat, blue bean-baggy thing on the table. It would become my personal pod, soon to be molded precisely to my body in the correct position for treatment. This would make it easier for them to replicate my position for each treatment. Just hop into the pod, and I'd be almost ready.

But first … ah, yes, the balloon. My very first. I am sad to say I never actually saw this special balloon, and don't even know what color it was. But as we progressed with this procedure, the color became less of a concern to me. Here is how it went between me and the radiation therapist (RT):

> RT: Okay, Mr. Nelson, please roll onto your left side for me.
>
> Me: Like this?
>
> RT: That's fine. Now, how's everything going for you back there today?

I would hear this question 39 more times, prior to each treatment. The therapists are religious about asking. To those of us who completed proton treatment, questions beginning with "How's it going" will never be heard in quite the same way again, and will likely always send a brief anticipatory chill down our spine.

Me:	What? What exactly does that mean?
RT:	Well, are you experiencing any unusual discomfort of any kind today in your rectal area? Hemorrhoids acting up maybe, or other irritation?
Me:	I see. No, this is just a lovely day for me "back there." Have at it.
RT:	Great. I'm going to insert the balloon now, slowly, and it should be painless, so be sure to let me know if you feel any discomfort.
Me:	All right. I'm sure it will feel just great, but I'll keep you posted.
RT:	Here we go … and … and … and … and … done. Okay so far?
Me:	So far, so good.

I then discovered that my initial fear of accidentally pushing the balloon back out was unfounded. Once the balloon is fully inserted, it is beyond the muscles that have the push-it-out reflex.

RT:	Now I'm going to fill the balloon with a saline solution. It will feel cold, and you will have a feeling of fullness, and again, there should be no pain.
Me:	Sounds terrific.
RT:	Here it comes …

The sensation of the balloon filling is not terrific. It was indeed cold, and when the balloon was just about full, I did feel a bit of brief, but easily tolerable pain. I think it was partly due to not relaxing, which I later learned to do (39 times provides plenty of opportunity to practice), and then rarely felt pain or discomfort most of the time.

Me:	Whoa! Hey there, that kind of hurts.
RT:	Okay, I'm finished. That discomfort should pass very quickly.
Me:	Yes, I'm fine now. Thank you.
RT:	Now, slowly roll over onto your back and make yourself comfortable.

This was easier said than done, and of course, they were doing the saying and I was doing the doing. I had no experience rolling around with an inflated balloon up my butt (and for that matter, neither did the therapists), so it required a new kind of effort and skill to complete this roll. Making myself comfortable was pretty much a lost cause, but I made a reasonable effort.

The table on which I was comfortably relaxing was part of a CT scanner, and for the next segment of my simulation I would be moved in and out of the scanner for brief looks at my prostate's position, with the help of the gold markers. This scanning was uneventful. No injections, no iodine, no scary tubes. Just in and out, in and out. Once the therapists were satisfied with my position, the air was sucked out of the blue beanbag pod[6] as they pressed its sides up against my legs, buttocks, and feet. In this process the pod becomes rigid, precisely shaped to my correctly positioned body. I would mount this pod 39 more times.

While I was lying on the pod, they shone a horizontal red laser light on both of my hips, and with a heavy magic marker, drew an X to mark the spots where the light hit me. Later, during actual treatments, they would shine the beam again and adjust my position in my pod until the beam hit the marks. Is this a high-tech operation, or what?

---

[6] By the way, although it is a blue pod, it is a green operation. The pods are recycled once treatments are complete. However, if you should ever become a proton prostate patient, you'll be happy to know the balloons are not recycled.

A clear round bandage was placed on top of each X, and I was instructed to make sure the X and the bandage remained until I returned in a month or so for treatments. I could shower, but I could not rub the X away. I'd like to add that this bandage was amazing. It did not even begin to come loose during the following weeks-in-waiting, and there was no irritation of any kind from it. But ultimately when the time came to remove it, it came off painlessly and effortlessly. I was impressed with the bandage. Maybe I'm easily impressed, but details do matter.

During the scanning and pod creation I was informed that my bladder had not filled, in which case, said the RT, they had three options: more water, more time, or both. They opted to give me another fifteen minutes of holding my pee (and my breath), and were then satisfied that 15 ounces and 45 minutes was the right formula for me. The usual deal is 15 ounces and 30 minutes, but it seems about twenty percent of the guys need more time, more water, or both. I knew one unlucky fellow who needed to drink 3 glasses of water (about 24 ounces) and wait an hour. I was relatively fortunate.

So now my bladder was full, the balloon was in place, the pod was created, and I was fully calibrated for treatments. I was asked to roll onto my left side again, and the balloon was emptied and removed. Now, I must tell you this is one of the strangest phenomena I've ever experienced. On the way in, the balloon felt like the six inches of its actual size. But on the way out it felt like a ten foot anaconda. It just seemed to keep coming, and coming, and coming. Other guys have confirmed this mind-blowing paradox. I still don't understand it.

At this point I was feeling tired and light-headed, which I assumed was because it had been a busy day, and I had some reflux which I assumed was due to being on my back. As I'll explain soon, neither assumption was correct. You will likely experience neither, so don't worry. It's part of my story, but probably won't be part of yours.

The final step was to take 3D pictures of my prostate so a brass aperture[7] and Lucite lens could be manufactured especially for me.

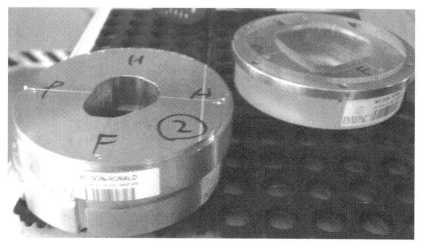

I was led into the adjoining room and hopped up (in truth, I wasn't doing much hopping at that point, but it sounds more cheerful, doesn't it?) onto the open MRI table. An *open* MRI does not involve a tube. It is more like a sandwich in which you are the meat. There was machinery above and below me, but not around me. Claustrophobia was not a significant issue. The issues for me were dizziness, reflux, and some anxiety resulting from that, not from the MRI. I do remember thinking how odd it was that this MRI was causing such sensations, but as it turned out, the MRI was not the culprit. You'll be fine.

After about fifteen minutes of the MRI, I was done. I would have jumped for joy, except I felt lousy. I thanked everyone, got dressed, went back into the lobby, and told Lucy to please head directly back to the apartment. I knew things were not going well. This was unfortunate, as it was Wednesday and we had planned to attend the free luncheon if time permitted. The timing was right, but I was not. Thankfully, I had managed to complete all of Phase 2 before my imminent meltdown, so the timing could have been worse.

---

[7] Greenies will again be pleased to know the brass is later melted and recycled. The Lucite cannot be reused, and is given to patients as a parting gift and treasured souvenir that can be used as an attractive candy dish.

I spent the rest of the day in the apartment, sitting in the recliner with an upset stomach, total loss of appetite, dry mouth, furry tongue, and eventually some rather violent primal vomiting. As a bonus, I later developed a red-dotted rash on my face. I was totally immobilized and ever-so-thankful Lucy was there to take care of me and figure out what to do. She called my case manager at around noon, who suggested giving it a little time to see if it passed. That is when the vomiting and rash began, and at 4:00 Lucy called again. This time Casey recommended a walk-in emergency place nearby (just in case), and instructed me to stop taking the Flagyl component of the antibiotic brew I was given to prevent infection from the gold marker procedure. Guess what! I am allergic to Flagyl. So now I know.

By 5:15 I was feeling a little more energy and the symptoms had begun to subside a bit. Lucy went shopping for some chicken soup, Jell-O, and Saltines so I could hopefully eat something. The only food I'd eaten that day was an English muffin before going to the Institute.

Our original plan was to celebrate completion of the simulation by attending the Wednesday luncheon, or maybe going out for a steak dinner at Ruth's Chris. We were hoping to pack up, head for home, and wake up in our own bed Thursday morning. This was not going to happen. I was not up to the trip and was just hoping I'd be well enough to travel in the morning.

Thursday I awoke tired, brain-dead, with a slightly upset stomach, but more than eager to go home. I was ready to tackle the five hour interstate highway drive, although the holiday traffic (it was December) would be no fun. Without pushing myself, we packed up and were on the road by about noon. Lucy has since told me she was ready and eager to put a little steam into the packing effort and leave hours earlier, but exercised great restraint, resisting the urge to use her own technique on my butt to get me moving more quickly. She was most kind to let me move at my own comfortable pace.

We were home at 5:00, December 23rd, and the pace would now only accelerate. We were expecting a houseful of holiday guests (family and extended family) the very next day, but did not have the benefit of the day between Florida and our guests' arrival that we had initially reserved to prepare for the visit. So as soon as we were home, we (by we, I mean Lucy) had to shift gears and scramble to do what should have been done the day before.

While Lucy shopped and readied the guest rooms, I unpacked and had plenty of time to think about how I would soon be repacking for a two-month return visit to Florida, without Lucy. It just didn't seem possible, but I knew it was coming. But coming even sooner, like starting the next day, were my four daughters, three grandkids, two sons-in-law, two boyfriends of daughters, and two parents (whom we had not previously met) of one of those boyfriends. I needed to conserve energy to focus on being a cheerful host and helpful husband.

The visit was great, and not at all about cancer. I was upbeat, truly, and I know all of my daughters were reassured that I was and would be fine. I was learning that the cancer experience was much more about them than me. I had done my research, seen the facility, spoken with other patients, and earned the confidence that my plan was going to have a positive result. But to others, the big "C" word is ominous, and they worry. So the visit was well-timed for them, and was an effective distraction for me. They did not all visit on the same days, and the overlapping comings and goings brought us into the new year, with just a couple of weeks left before I headed south.

After the holidays, I worked a couple of normal weeks while preparing for the long haul in Jacksonville. I bought a laptop to facilitate working remotely, made a packing list, and tied up a few loose ends. As departure day approached, the experience became increasingly surreal. I did not (and do not) like being away from home. I'm a homebody, and I surely don't like being apart from Lucy. In fact, I think the upcoming trip would represent the longest away game I have played, and certainly my longest separation from Lucy. But it would not be indefinite. Two months, and done. Others have done it. We could do it. And then life would return to normal.

As it turned out, life would not return to the prior normal. I would have a new normal. People would call me a cancer survivor (woo hoo!), and I would be hanging around a lot with guys who had, have, or were concerned they might possibly someday have prostate cancer, providing my sage advice to newbies. And in my new normal I would write a book.

Southward, Ho!

I worked a full time schedule right up until the big day arrived. Monday (January 17, 2011) was Martin Luther King Day, so Lucy and I had a full day off from work together. Nice. She had to work Tuesday and Wednesday, and I had to do some big-time packing Tuesday to be ready to head south Wednesday morning. We were in a daze, with nothing in our history that compared to what we faced, and no way to judge exactly how we'd feel. We just plowed ahead toward my inevitable departure.

Early Wednesday morning we said our goodbyes, and then Lucy left for work. I finished packing and hit the road at 10:15, with my Pacifica (not a minivan) crammed full of all the gear I could squeeze into it. I do not travel light. I like my stuff. I even brought my gigantic computer monitor to use with my laptop. Of course, all of my coffee paraphernalia came with me, as did my Harmony Sovereign acoustic guitar, and my Kindle e-reader. At least I could sit around drinking good coffee, making mediocre music or reading a crappy book. That's basically what I do anyway, so it would feel a bit like home. In fact, at this very moment I'm sitting around drinking excellent coffee, writing a mediocre book. Wait—no—it's a great book!

I live in an extraordinarily beautiful, peaceful, rural part of the midlands of South Carolina, a heavenly secluded spot no one stumbles upon, on a private pond, down a dead end dirt road. I love it here, and I love living here with Lucy. Leaving, I knew, would be one of the toughest parts of this adventure. Knowing this, I did not plan to return home until the job was complete. I just didn't think I wanted to repeat the leaving home experience. Also, driving five hours to spend little more than a day at home, just to leave again right away and drive five hours to return to Jacksonville seemed like what would probably be an exhausting, unfulfilling proposition. So this was goodbye for two months. Lucy was understanding and supportive of this decision, which essentially made her responsible for any visiting that would occur during the next couple months.

By 10:00 I was nearly finished packing, ready to leave. I'll admit to being close to tears, with butterflies in my stomach and wobbly knees. This was like nothing I had ever done. I know, I'm a wuss. There. I admit it. As I write this now, Topher, my son-in-law, is on a naval aircraft carrier half way around the world from his wife, daughter, and unborn child in California, and will be gone for six months or more with limited communication of any kind. I'll have my cell phone, email, Skype, and will be only 300 miles away, by land. So yes, again, I am a wuss, and he is a real man. But we are each fighting our own very different battles. Oh, yes, and he is twenty-seven years old. I'm sixty-one. I don't know why that matters, but don't I deserve some kind of a wuss handicap for age?

At 10:15 I was on the road, which happened to be mucky, slushy, and filthier than usual as a result of an unusual southern snowstorm the prior week. We had been completely snowed in until just days before, and if I had been scheduled for Florida even a week earlier than I was, I would have been unable to drive out on the only road to and from our house, even with the awesome power of a 2007 Pacifica. So the timing worked out, and off I went with a heavy heart, but a determined mind.

I stopped at a quick car wash to clean off the snowy filth and to gas up for the trip. As it turned out, my car remained clean for the entire two months in Jacksonville. Along with everything else, a clean car was a new experience for me. Driving to my house requires traveling a dirt road that is usually bone dry, and by the time I arrive home my car is invariably covered in dust. I've lived here for eleven years now, and that's how long it's been since I've attempted to have a clean car for even a day. Every time I saw my car in Jacksonville, my reaction was: "Aha, so *that's* what color it is!"

The drive was uneventful. I arrived at Third and Main at 3:40 and spent the rest of the day unpacking and settling in. Third and Main was not new to me. We had stayed there for the Phase 1, Phase 2 visit, so this was at least one part of the trip that was a known commodity. It's a great place to stay, and in a small way I felt I had returned to my home away from home.

Now the trick was to get a good night's sleep, and to be ready for my first proton treatment the next day. I could hardly wait.

Phase 3: Treatments

Thursday, January 20th. My first treatment day. I woke up without an alarm at around 7:00, went through my coffee ritual, toasted an English muffin for breakfast, exercised in Third and Main's exercise room, showered, and planned a shopping trip to Radio Shack, Lowes, and Publix. This was the beginning of my effort to create a temporary "new normal" lifestyle away from home.

I was originally scheduled to see Dr. Candor at 4:30, and to have my first proton blast at 6:30, but those times were changed to 5:00 and 7:00. Then, when I called at 1:00 to reconfirm, I was told to arrive at 4:00 because Dr. Candor leaves at 5:00 on Thursday. I would need time to check in, do some more paperwork (after all, a day without paperwork is like a … whatever), and see Dr. Candor. These scheduling issues of this first day are not typical, they reassured me.

I easily arrived on time, being only five minutes from the Institute, parked in the gated private lot, politely greeted the smiling security guard at the entrance, walked cautiously up to the reception desk, and identified myself to the pretty, gregarious, and most welcoming afternoon/evening receptionist who loves to munch pork rinds, among other goodies. I'll protect her identity and affectionately call her Sally.

Sally:	Hello there, Mr. Nelson! Welcome! Let me find your accessory for you.
Me:	My what?
Sally:	Your accessory.
Me:	What's an accessory?
Sally:	Oh, you know! Like I wear necklaces and bracelets to accessorize? This will be *your* accessory for the next couple months. Put it around your neck and wear it while you are here.
Me:	Okay, thanks. Very stylish accessory.

Sally: Yes. It's your ID. You just wave it under the scanner over there as soon as you arrive each day, and that lets them know in the treatment room that you are here and ready. Your name should appear on the monitor near the scanner, and when you see it, press Enter. Go ahead, do it now!

So I waved the card under the scanner and scanned myself in for the first time, just like the self-checkout at Lowe's. Only this time I really was self-checking myself, and I was checking in, not out. I saw my name on the screen (certainly a thrill) and pressed Enter. Never forget to press Enter. If you don't press Enter, they won't know you're there and you won't be treated, and your trip to Jacksonville will have been for nothing. So press Enter.

Sally then used her super-secret under-the-desk button to open the "authorized personnel only" sliding glass doors to her right and just behind her, directing me to enter and have a seat. This was the doorway to the inner waiting area just outside the treatment rooms, some offices, and several small examination rooms where case managers routinely interview and doctors periodically see the patients and sometimes share a DRE or a barium cocktail.

I then learned the various steps I would experience once each week during treatment. I was weighed, my blood pressure and pulse were taken, and then I was escorted to one of those small rooms. I was again greeted by my case manager, Casey, with whom I'd had the pleasure of working last month during my poking and prodding phase. First, we reminisced about my Flagyl meltdown. Ah, those were the days. Then she gave me the twenty questions I came to think of as the Weekly Pee and Poop Report. I don't know how she could ask these questions with a straight face, but she did. I certainly could not answer them with a straight face. Here, you try it:

So, Mr. Nelson, any pain while urinating? Any blood? Leakage? How often? How many times at night? Slow to start? Strong stream? Do you completely empty your bladder? How far can you squirt? Can you write your name in the snow? Pee while standing on your head?

With your eyes closed? Without missing the target?

There was a similar set of interview questions regarding pooping, but I will spare you the details of that one. Use your imagination. You'll probably be correct. Curiously, they did not seem to be interested in my weekly sexual performance. No questions about that at all. Too bad. You could construct a captivating, probing interview script on that topic.

Then I saw Dr. Candor, and I remember nothing about that meeting except that he no longer had a cold and his voice sounded pleasantly normal. As long as nothing is going haywire, the weekly interview with the oncologist is mostly just touching bases. It's an opportunity to discuss issues, just in case, but there seems to be no other agenda. Still, this works well. I liked seeing a doctor now and then. It gave me a feeling of confidence, like knowing the Wizard of Oz is reassuringly behind the curtain, making things work as they should, watching out for me.

However, I will take the opportunity now to say that although I liked seeing my doctor, it was even more comforting and reassuring to know there was a whole team of experts planning, overseeing, and administering my care. From the security guard to the receptionists, office staff, nurses, doctors, physicists, and the crackerjack team of radiation therapists treating me daily, I was in good hands. I liked the fact that my treatment did not depend heavily on the expertise of a single individual, as it would, for example, with surgery. My proton radiation treatment was a carefully orchestrated symphony, and if one player hit a bad note, another would correct him. The checks and double-checks built into this system promised a consistent result from day to day, and patient to patient. It is impressive, and I liked it.

After seeing Dr. Candor I was ushered back into the main outer lobby, and took a seat in the large semi-circle of easy chairs. Seated next to me was a man with an accessory of his own (aha, he's a patient, I brilliantly surmised), diddling around with an iPad. After a few minutes, he took the initiative and introduced himself. It was his second day. We exchanged stories, and he related to me that he had somehow received five gold marker implants, one more than the expected four. This necessitated a repeat of his simulation phase.

Well, I was certainly off to a better start. I had only the expected four markers. No extras, and no re-dos for me.

As my appointed treatment time of 7:00 pm approached, one of the RTs (radiation therapists) greeted me in the lobby and instructed me to "empty and drink." Again, this does not refer to my wallet and booze at the local bar. Here it means "pee your heart out" and then "imbibe an ungodly amount of water you'll have to hold for what will seem like the rest of your life." Sure. I can do that.

I went into what would become one of my favorite, most frequented rest rooms—the main lobby men's room—took my stance at the urinal, and had no difficulty emptying. But then, I had not received any radiation yet. I did notice a towel on the floor below the urinal, and after some contemplation, I decided it was a nice touch. Many men's rooms could use similar attention, but this one in particular, I learned, was most often used by guys who had unpredictable, sometimes uncontrollable streams that were not always accurately aimed, through no fault of their own. Through no fault of *our* own, I should say. I was one of those guys, or would soon become one. It's usually a temporary condition, and reassuring to know the folks at Florida Proton were aware of it, acknowledged it, and met even this small challenge head on. Kudos!

Next stop, the water cooler, where you'll find stacks and stacks of eight ounce Styrofoam cups. Two of those babies, please, down the hatch. The water is extremely cold. After all, it's a water cooler. It's too cold for some guys, and I've seen them mix some hot water (provided for making hot chocolate, mostly for visitors) to raise the temperature, but not me. I can take it straight, and cold. I'm a real man.

Having emptied, I had time to sit for a little while, anticipating the big event. My debut performance. The fancy white polka dotted gown, my comfy blue pod, the balloon, and (hopefully) a little proton radiation to make it all worthwhile. Finally, an RT arrived to escort me to the dressing room. Just like simulation. I knew exactly how to remove my shoes, pants, and undies. Yes, I did. I crammed all of that and my hefty man purse into the locker, locked it, put the stretchy key bracelet on my wrist, took a deep breath or two, and pulled back the curtain. This time I refrained from shouting "TA DA," opting for a more dignified opening performance.

I was then reminded to wait in the dressing room until retrieved by an RT. This is in deference to the privacy of the prior patient as they exit, to protect their identity and their … their hiney, usually at least partially hanging out the backside of the gown. There is just no way to tie the gown's two sets of meager little laces adequately to prevent some overexposure. I guess that's probably the whole point of the gown design, after all: easy access to the necessary gateway. So the prior patient exits the treatment room and either bolts full steam ahead for the bathroom directly across from the dressing room and quickly closes the door, or enters the other of the two side-by-side dressing rooms and closes the curtain. At that point it's deemed safe for me to reveal myself and enter the treatment room unseen, with my predecessor anonymously out of sight. A therapist retrieves me and leads me into the treatment room.

This concern with our vanity is refreshing, but later becomes unnecessary. We soon lose all humility, and most of us couldn't care less who sees what, or who can identify us. The above routine just kind of falls apart of its own accord. I was often preceded by a sweet little old granny-type lady, who clearly had no interest in hiding from me. We exchanged smiles and nods as she left, and I entered. She saw some of mine, and I saw some of hers, hers not especially interesting to me, and vice versa, I'm sure.

By the way, prostate cancer is not the only type of cancer treated at Florida Proton, and granny probably did not have prostate cancer, even though her uniform was the same as mine. In addition to grannies and old men, there were a surprising number of children being treated for brain tumors, and this was a sobering sight. The children were generally far less uptight about treatment than we wise old grownups, but their parents clearly understood the risks and the stakes, and were ever so grateful that our health care system made this advanced high-tech treatment available. The families here from abroad were especially thankful for the opportunity.

I didn't always follow granny. I sometimes followed prostate guys who would warn me that they had unfortunately used the last of the lubricant, leaving none to grease the way for my balloon. So sorry. Ha ha. No problem, I quipped. I brought some WD-40 just in case. Ha ha. Then, I would repeat this lame exchange with guy who followed me. We are all so clever. But vain? Not so much. Not any more. In addition to curing cancer, this process cures vanity.

The radiation therapists seem to sense exactly when a patient has passed through vanity's exit door. At that point, they continue to escort you back to the dressing room, but then pretty much leave you to figure out what to do next on your own. After all, most of us prostate guys get 39 times to figure it out, and we're pretty smart fellows, on average. The RT eventually stops making the trip from the treatment room to the dressing room to retrieve patients. They just call from the treatment room, "Okay, Mr. Nelson, you can come in whenever you're ready." And in I would march, with a spring in my step, butt hanging out for the entire world to see, if anyone was interested.

Now the real fun began. My special time. For the next 15-30 minutes it would be all about me. As I entered the treatment room there was almost always music playing, courtesy of the RT *team du jour*. Sometimes a little Motown mix, sometimes Sinatra, sometimes … whatever. If I wanted, I could bring my own mix CD, but I liked the variety they provided and preferred to be surprised, exploring new genres of music as part of my experience, some I never knew existed. At the time, I was sixty years old. I estimate their average age to be about 17, so of course they knew about some music I didn't. Most of it was pretty enjoyable.

Now we need to be serious. The next phase is all about security, accuracy, checks, and cross-checks. Upon entering the room it was my responsibility—that's right, *my* job—to check three different computer monitors along the wall to my right, at the front of the room, to make sure it was my name and my picture displayed. After all, I know me, right? I handed my ID card to an RT who scanned it. I was bar-coded, as all Americans will be eventually. The scanning confirmed that the brass aperture and Lucite lens, also bar-coded and scanned, matched mine.

Once everyone was satisfied that it was really me (not someone pretending to be me just so they could get some proton radiation) and really my stuff, then I could climb the little step ladder to easily mount the table—the *slab*. Oops, one more thing: make sure my name is on the pod. I wouldn't want to cram myself into the wrong pod, now would I? I liked my pod, custom fit to me. This was truly the royal treatment. My name was everywhere. Me, me, me.

So then, holding the 15 ounces of water I drank 45 minutes to an hour ago, I climbed into my pod, making sure my stocking feet were snugly pressed into the bottom, just so. Ahhhhh. Better than Select-Comfort. Who needs a Sleep Number when you have your own high-tech pod? At first the RTs would instruct me to roll onto my left side, but it didn't take me too many treatments to learn to predict this instruction, and like a well-trained puppy I would just roll over on my own.

At first I wasn't sure what to do with my legs and knees to make the balloon's upcoming journey as uneventful as possible, but eventually I figured out a position that worked. I suspect this varies with different people. Your balloon-ready posture might be different than mine. No problem, though. There'll be plenty of chances to experiment. If you don't get it exactly right today, make adjustments tomorrow. This is your new life. My new life. Accommodating balloons up my butt. Your butt. Whatever.

Then came the question I vaguely recalled from simulation, the question that will never again sound the same to me. It was part of the ritual. The exact phrasing varied, but it amounted to this:

> *How's everything going for you back there*
> *today, Mr. Nelson?*

Of course, "back there" referred to my butt hole. The question was an invitation for me to describe any back door distress—hemorrhoids, rashes, itching, burning, pain, throbbing, little creatures dancing, lost items rolling around—that might make the balloon insertion less enjoyable than usual. Typically, everything was going fine back there, and we moved right along to the main event. Sometimes I took the occasion to attempt some humor. I am sure the RTs genuinely appreciated my jokes, and I'm equally certain all my jokes were new creations, never heard before. The RTs would often say, "Good one, Mr. Nelson. I never heard that before."

Now here's an interesting oddity. I was about to have a balloon shoved up my butt, but that is not what concerned me most. I had a reasonable handle on that, especially after a little practice. But what produced greater anxiety at this moment were two possibilities: I could lose the liquid (i.e., pee in my pod), and I could pass gas in a most embarrassing way. In either case I knew I would be unable to successfully pass the buck as I so adeptly do in restaurants and other public places, declaring "it wasn't me" while pointing at an unsuspecting bystander. There were no bystanders here. I was alone, on stage. It was me. Undeniably. I never did lose control of my bladder while on the slab, and I think I did a respectable job avoiding adding any ominous sound effects or unwelcome aromas into the atmosphere. But if anyone were to ask me to identify the most difficult part of receiving proton radiation therapy, this would be it. Not peeing, not flatulating. That was the challenge.

I was ready for the balloon. The RT would say something like, "Okay, here we go," and in just a minute or so I'd hear the update that it was in, and the saline would be injected to inflate it. Some of the RTs tended to be a little quick with the saline injection, and I found it helpful if they took that part a little slower, so I reminded them of that each time, and they were always politely accommodating. Nice and easy, just for me.

A little more detail about the balloon: I should make it clear that this balloon is not a party balloon, although they are often depicted that way. It is a high-tech medical item. It has a depth calibrator so they know precisely how far it must be inserted each time without guessing (determined during Phase 2 simulation). Better than asking each time, "Hey, Mr. Nelson, is that far enough?" It has two tubes: one to attach the saline syringe, and another with an exit-only release valve allowing any gas in the intestine to escape rather than compress back into the intestine, bloating it. This gas release system is ingenious. There is great concern about gaseousness because gas in the intestine can make the prostate move more than it already does. Thus the concern for a gas-free diet, and the presence of Gas-X tablets in my medicine chest. But gas is far less of a concern with these improved balloons with the gas release tube, a clever touch. Better safe than sorry.

My balloon:

Party balloon:

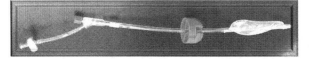

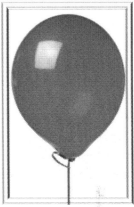

So with the saline / gas-release tube hanging between my legs like a little tail, I slowly rolled over trying not to squeeze my butt muscles. It wouldn't matter if I did, but it just didn't seem right to me. The balloon stays in without my help, and there is no way I know of to accidentally squeeze it out, but it somehow seemed incumbent upon me to keep my muscles down there relaxed. At least it gave me something to do, or not do, and it's not as easy as you might think. It is true that the less activity in that area, the better, to keep the prostate stationary. This is very important because it's harder to hit a moving target. So I tried not to squeeze my buns, not to move, and not to pee, which about sums up my active role in this event.

Allow me to digress for a minute, and say that these highly skilled and professional radiation therapists are coincidentally a terrific looking (by terrific, I mean "hot") bunch of youngsters. Even the guys. I doubt this is officially part of the hiring criteria, but it certainly doesn't hurt that it worked out that way. I have my personal favorite, of course, but I will not identify her. This is a tell-all book, but not that kind. However, I will admit that from time to time I have found myself wondering whether I might not need to return to Florida for just a little more radiation.

As I now more objectively contemplate this bizarre daily scenario, I am reminded that you can never predict what life has in store for you, and some of it is indeed bizarre, even farfetched. If someone had said to me 30 years ago: "Ron, I know you'll find this hard to believe, but 30 years from now you will be surrounded every day by beautiful, smiling, caring young women (along with some fine looking young men) half your age, taking turns putting things up your butt, ever so gently," I would have died laughing, maybe literally, and prostate cancer might never have been an issue. But there I was, in precisely that situation. Life is strange, is it not?

We have reached an appropriate time to introduce a new word: *gantry*. This refers to the giant three story structure into which the table and I are moved, from which the proton beam will come. For convenience, the treatment room itself is referred to as the gantry, but it's really just the structure at the back of the room. At the time of my treatment there were three: the yellow, red, and blue gantries. They are not actually colored that way, but it's more fun than calling them gantry #1, #2, and #3, and the colors are reminiscent of festive balloon colors. They could have named the gantries after animals, cartoon characters, or past presidents I suppose, but let's not be silly. Yellow, red, and blue.

For the record, I was assigned to the blue gantry. However, the RTs are not tied to a specific gantry. There is no permanent blue gantry staff, for example. They work in teams of three, and a given team works in the same gantry on the same shift (morning or evening) for a week, sometimes more. Then they are switched to another area to gain expertise not only with the proton beam and balloons, but also CT scans, MRIs, PET scans, and even IMRT (yes, UFPTI can use photon radiation when appropriate, too). Periodically the director of this operation scrambles the teams around so each RT never works with the same partners for too long, kind of like a square dance. My understanding is that this keeps them more alert, and less likely to become set in their ways or complacent. No bonding is allowed amongst the RTs. Don't get too comfortable; you'll be on a new team very soon. Makes sense to me. Keeps everyone focused.

Now, back to the gantry. It's hard to describe a gantry, but I'll give it a shot. It's overwhelmingly impressive to see it first-hand and up close. Imagine standing in front of a clothes dryer with its front door and front panel removed, so you can see the entire inside drum. Now imagine the diameter of the drum being three stories high. The drum turns, just like a clothes dryer, but very slowly. Protruding from the curved wall of the drum is a proton beam gun, connected to the cyclotron in the super-secret back room where the protons are generated, shot through the gun, and ultimately into the patient (me). The drum rotates to reposition the direction of the gun, and it can move a full 360 degrees around me. On the flat back wall of the drum are several retractable X-ray units. When not in use, they retract and become flush with the back wall. When needed, they come forward sticking out into the drum. It's quite a contraption.

The table on which I was comfortably relaxing in my pod is just outside the gantry, suspended over the regular flat floor in the treatment room, and I was initially positioned with my feet pointing into the gantry, just outside of it at its edge. Once I was comfortable in my pod, balloon in butt, the therapists carefully lined me up with horizontal red laser lights that should hit the magic marker Xs drawn on my hips during simulation. The RTs physically rolled me a little this way or that, until the lasers precisely hit their mark. This is an important step toward ensuring that I am positioned correctly.

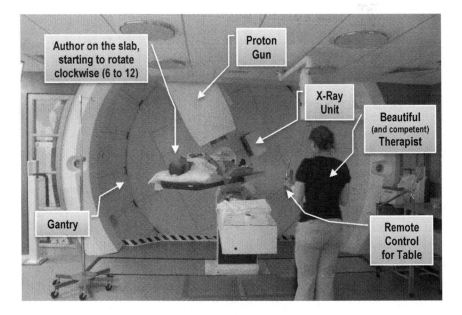

The table then slowly swung around clockwise, like the hand of clock with my feet at the center, moving my head from the 6 to the 12. Having moved 180 degrees, my feet remained in about the same place, but my head and most of my body were inside the gantry. I was on the table suspended in the drum, head near the back, feet near the treatment room. There was sometimes a feeling of dizziness or vertigo in this position, especially when the drum began to rotate, but it's not strong and most of us proton guys adapted quickly.

The gantry rotated to move the proton gun to my left side one day, my right the next. Alternating sides extended the recovery time for each side to 48 hours. Next, the X-ray units came out of the back wall and extended directly above me, below me, and/or on one side. A low energy X-ray detected my gold markers, and projected this on a monitor for an RT who used a remote control to adjust the table position in extremely small increments to perfectly align me and my markers with the required imagery obtained during simulation, so the beam would hit the prostate precisely. They then easily inserted my copper aperture and Lucite lens into the gun so the beam would be perfectly shaped in 3D to the shape of my prostate.

With me and the table precisely aligned, the X-ray units retracted into the back wall. The RTs then rang a bell that sounds like a doorbell chime (a single "ding"). This was their way of announcing they were going to retire to their private control room on the other side of the front wall to sip coffee and play computer solitaire, leaving me alone with my private thoughts, staring upward into the gantry.

This upward staring is hypnotic. The compulsion to study the tiniest details of the gantry's construction is irresistible. Where are the screws? How many? Where are the seams? In the blue gantry there was something that looked like a piece of duct tape stuck on the gantry wall. I knew that piece of duct tape intimately, and wondered about it every time I saw it. But duct tape is comforting. It saves lives. Remember Apollo 13?

The gantry then rotated again to precisely aim the gun at either my left or right hip, and then the gun protruded a little more, coming close to me, but not in an alarming way. I could hear various sounds throughout all of the above steps, and during the coming weeks those sounds would become comforting and predictable. I heard the clanging of the aperture and lens being inserted by the RT. I heard (and felt) the table adjusting in tiny increments. I heard the RTs walking. I heard the doorbell ding. I heard whirring sounds of various pitches. And I tried to figure out what it all meant, and more specifically, I wanted to know when the beam started shooting me.

But alas, there is no indicator announcing when the beam starts, so I could only guess, and I badly wanted to know. I wanted to know this for no reason other than I thought I should know. There is absolutely no sensation whatsoever while the beam shoots, so it hardly matters, but still, I wanted to know. But I could not. I tried to correlate the sounds with the start/end of the beam, but was never able to do so successfully. To make it even harder to guess, the source of the beam (the back-room cyclotron) can only feed protons to one gantry at a time, so sometimes the blue gantry gets the beam right away, and other times there might be a few minutes of waiting until another gantry finishes with it. Outside the room there is indeed a "Beam On" sign that lights up (like "On Air" in a radio studio), but that didn't help me on the table. This was frustrating, and I was inevitably just a little surprised when I heard the RTs re-enter the room, the first sign that I was done. But it did give me something to think about as I mentally grooved to the music the RTs left playing on their CD player.

The beam only lasts about a minute, they told me, although I had no idea when it started or ended. But soon enough I heard footsteps and more clanking as my lens and aperture were removed. Those sounds became the eagerly anticipated signal that I was on my way out. Then, as the table began to swing me back counterclockwise from 12 to 6 on the imaginary clock, one of the RTs invited me to roll onto my left side again and raise my right knee. The lucky therapist then drained the saline (*ahhhhhh*) and slowly removed the balloon. Once the RTs were confident I was sufficiently experienced with this exit procedure, they would often begin balloon extraction while the table was still in motion. They were always eager to remove the balloon, and I suppose I was, too. They were also understandably aware of the tight schedule they must keep, and getting the balloon out facilitates getting me out so they could shout to the next guy to "come on in whenever you're ready, Mr. so-and-so!" We all became very chummy.

Now let's see if you were paying attention in the earlier chapter on simulation: What is six inches long on the way in, but ten feet long on the way out? Yes! The balloon. You *were* paying attention! Only prostate cancer proton patients can answer this from firsthand knowledge, and all of us can answer without hesitation. The withdrawal of the balloon is not uncomfortable, but is always totally unnerving, quite memorable, and unquestionably mind-blowing. A great climax to a wonderful experience.

I climbed out of my pod, stepped down from the table using the little step stool, adjusted my gown a bit, and met one the RTs on the opposite side of the room near the array of computer monitors on the front wall, where I had checked in just minutes earlier. They removed the little appointment card from the pocket of my so-called accessory, and wrote my next treatment time on the scheduling grid. You might assume, as I did initially, that patients would be assigned a standard treatment time, the same time every day, but you'd be wrong. You are given only one appointment, the next one, following each treatment, and it is rarely the same time as the previous one.

The fact is, treatment times are a premium commodity. If this were prison, you could trade cigarettes for times. Patients vie for the best times, which most consider to be the early morning slots. The reason for this is simple: if your treatment is over before breakfast, you are free for the rest of the day to play. Many patients are retired and like to play golf. You might recall that Jacksonville is in Florida. They have golf there. Some guys are accompanied by their wives, so they have to go shopping. They have stores in Florida, too. Some guys (like me) don't play golf, don't have the daily pleasure of their wives' company, and are not retired. So I worked via remote connection to my office back home, gallantly putting in about half of my usual hours. Remember, I was busy fighting cancer. So I explored Jacksonville, went to parks, museums, met my new friends for lunch or dinner, and had a relaxing, low stress time, even without golf, even without Lucy. It was not bad at all.

The least popular times are the evening ones, or even the late afternoon slots, but I preferred them. I settled into a comfortable daily routine based on that kind of schedule, and I liked it. I would wake up with the sun, make a great pot of coffee and a light breakfast, and enjoy my meal while reading a good novel on my Kindle. Then I'd head down the hall at Third and Main to exercise, and sometimes chat with another patient doing the same. Then it was back to my apartment to shower and log into my office to work for an hour or two, maybe three. I would typically go out somewhere for lunch, maybe meeting one of my new proton buddies at one of the many excellent restaurants where we could dine outside and enjoy stimulating conversation, or maybe I'd go solo and leisurely read more of my novel. Then back to the apartment, work a while longer, and head over to the Institute for fun with balloons. Finally, back home (my temporary new one) I'd have dinner with TV, maybe work, maybe just catch up on email, usually spend quite a while

Skyping Lucy, and then go to bed. Not a bad routine, and I had little competition for the late afternoon time slots I wanted.

How are time slots allocated? Based on seniority. The newbies are given the late slots, and the closer you are to completion ("graduation"), the more likely you are to be scheduled whenever you prefer, usually early morning. The RTs do a highly respectable job of scheduling, and patients can give them a two hour preferred window for treatments. If you're hoping for the mornings, you can forget it until you're at least halfway through treatments. If you like afternoon or evening times, you'll have better luck sooner. If you have special circumstances like a concert, sporting event, visitors, plane schedules, or other time-sensitive considerations of a one-time nature, the RT will work with you to make that happen. They are always understanding and as helpful about this as possible.

So I was off the table, I'd been given my next appointment time, and I was done, much relieved that I had survived my first blast. I thanked the RTs, headed to the bathroom, got dressed, walked in a trance down the long hallway back to the lobby, and went directly out the door to my car, just a few steps away. I could pick up Chinese or Greek for dinner, or pop a Lean Cuisine into the microwave. I was happily relieved of any immediate concern about gaseousness or other gastronomic maladies because I would not be back on the slab for about a day. It was a feeling of release and relief. Freedom!

Weekends were even more liberating for eating. I always felt Friday dinner was a free pass to eat whatever I wanted. After all, I had all of Saturday, Sunday, and with my late appointments, most of Monday to recover from whatever damage I might do to my digestive system. And on occasion, damage I did indeed do. Fried food, spicy food, and usually too much food. Whatever. But it all worked out well in the end. Yes, that end.

One down, thirty-eight to go.

The 6 Stages of Balloonification

My wife Lucy is a psychologist, and a tiny bit of her ability and compulsion to *psychologize* has naturally rubbed off on me. This tendency gave me insight into the psychological aspect of a proton patient's relationship with the balloon. There are some clearly identifiable phases we experience, which I've labeled **The 6 Stages of Balloonification** and would like to share with you. Of course, there are variations and nuances depending on individual circumstances, but these six chronological phases are universal.

Stage 1: Disbelief

This occurs at the inevitable moment when we first learn about the use of the balloon in proton therapy, which is one of the most absurd sounding things imaginable at that moment. It can occur anywhere, at any time before your first treatment. This delightful tidbit of information might be first revealed to you by a former patient, your doctor, or someone else, but regardless of who breaks the news, the conversation between you and that guy might sound something like this:

That Guy:	Yeah, so, before you get the beam …
You:	Uh huh …
That Guy:	When you're on the table they, um, they like …
You:	Yes?
That Guy:	They roll you over onto your left side, and, um, and …
You:	And then …
That Guy:	They stick a balloon up your butt.
You:	*(pause … frown … look left … look right … look forward)* Uh … do **what** ???

| That Guy: | (*grinning*) Yeah, that's right. They stick a balloon up your butt. They grease it first, and then they *slooooooowly* slide it in and pump it full of water. They do this before each of your 39 treatments. (*smile, and nod once*) |
| You: | They do **what**??? **How** many times??? |

The general feeling is indeed disbelief, but even though at some level you soon realize that guy is not kidding, you still refuse to accept the bizarre notion, which leads to the next stage.

Stage 2: Denial

Between your 1st and 5th balloons, you continue to have a great deal of difficulty accepting that what that guy told you is true, even though you are already experiencing it daily. It all feels surreal, as if it is not really happening. It's just a dream. A weird, perverse dream.

You can easily identify patients at Balloonification Stage 2. They wear blank expressions, moving slowly in a zombie-like manner, looking directly at no one, and showing no sign of engagement with the real world. They are there, but not totally. They are in a daze of denial. But then …

Stage 3: Resignation / Acceptance

Beginning at the 6th balloon and continuing until the 18th, you basically surrender. You give up. Your attitude slides into one of: "Okay, fine. Have your way with me. Do what you need to do. Whatever." It's out of your hands, you know it, you can and must finally accept it, and you resign yourself to your fate.

Guys at Stage 3 are also easy to identify. They have regained some expression, have moderate interaction with other people, move a little more naturally, and might even smile now and then. They appear in most ways to be in a relatively normal state of mind. It is a survival tactic to accept what cannot be changed, and we do, and then just move on with life.

But then, the strangest of transformations occurs.

Stage 4: Enjoyment / Euphoria

Soon after the 18th balloon there is a marked change in outward behavior. We've adapted. More than adapted, we've embraced our new existence. Guys are almost giddy, always smiling and moving briskly. They literally march from the parking lot to the front door, high-fiving the security guard on the way into the Institute. They greet the receptionist with a smile and some clever banter. They wave to other guys across the room, often shouting, "Hey, buddy, how's it going!" or some such thing. They might not even bother to sit down, mingling with the crowd as if at a swank cocktail party. They move seamlessly from the water cooler to the jigsaw puzzle table, to the easy chairs, to the baby grand, and back to the reception desk for more witty repartee. They are in their element now, totally at ease, and they are thoroughly enjoying it.

This change in demeanor coincides with a change in attitude about the balloons. At this stage, guys have begun to look forward to the experience. Yes, we eventually learn to like the balloons and can hardly wait for the next one. Truth be told, that is the real reason we want those prized early morning treatment time slots. We just can't wait all day, now can we? We hop up onto the slab, sometimes bypassing the step stool, and we are on our left side in a flash with nary a command. "How's it going back there today, Mr. Nelson?" is a question that soothes my soul, and I reply: "I don't know, you tell me. You've got a better view. HA HA HA!" (the RTs genuinely appreciate that kind of humor).

Eventually treatment #39 occurs, or #28 for those on the short course (too bad, guys), and with it, Stage 5 arrives.

Stage 5: Separation Anxiety

Immediately or very soon after the final balloon, we have the unhappy realization that there will be no more balloons. We finish the treatment and reluctantly climb down from the table as the RTs applaud and congratulate us on completing the program. They do not write another appointment time on the back of our ID card. They will no longer be interested in *how it's going back there*. We are overwhelmed with sadness, and as we look around the gantry—*our* gantry—for the final time, we begin to face the fact that we will not see this fine crew of therapists again, because there are no second helpings of protons. We have had our fill, and they don't want us back. Although this may sound a bit melodramatic to you, it is pretty close to the truth.

Before I left Florida, I suggested to the folks at UFPTI that they offer an additional week of balloons for a fee of about $500. Balloons only, no radiation. Just hop on the table and get the balloon. The profits could be earmarked to benefit the children of all ages undergoing proton treatment. The service would help alleviate the separation anxiety of prostate patients, while the money would help the children. It would be a win-win scenario. I do not believe they have implemented this service yet.

Stage 6: Balloon Withdrawal

Within about four weeks following completion of therapy, after returning home, we regress. We hear voices in our head asking questions like, "Should I empty now? Time to drink? Roll over?" And then it dawns on us, again. We are done. Really. No more balloons, no more RTs, no more empty/drink. Done. And we feel the sadness again, the empty hole the balloon once filled. Time will eventually cure this, the final stage of Balloonification, and then life can resume anew, but we don't know that yet. It's a difficult stage.

Florida Proton should consider my other fund-raising idea to aid ex-patients at Stage 6. Why not let the RT of our choice make an on-site visit to our home for a week of homebound balloons? Why not! They could charge a hefty fee for that service, and proton children everywhere would rejoice! Brilliant!

I can only hope they have taken this suggestion under advisement, and are moving forward with it expeditiously. It's too late for me. I have finally recovered from stage 6, but we must think of the next guy, right?

Some have postulated that there might be a seventh stage of Balloonification, in which the former patient's memory begins playing tricks on him as he wonders whether the Florida experience was real or maybe only imagined. Who knows, it might have been a form of alien abduction, complete with the typical high-tech machinery and bodily probing associated with most documented real abductions. The abductee is transported elsewhere, examined, and returned with little evidence and often no clear memory of the experience.

Whether there is any truth to this stage-seven hypothesis remains to be seen.

Between Treatments

Each proton treatment takes about 30 minutes, start to finish, excluding time to "empty and drink." This leaves 23½ additional hours to fill each weekday. Subtracting eight hours for a hopefully good night's sleep, there remains … well let's just say there is a lot of time to fill, and there are numerous options for doing so. Some are provided by Florida Proton as part of their support for and encouragement of socialization among the patients. They want us to regard our visit as a positive experience—even a fun time—with many guys describing it as their "radiation vacation." Cute and clever. I wish I could lay claim to coining that popular phrase. Well, I guess I could, but I'd be lying.

So what do we do between treatments to kill all those hours? If you are a golfer, you play golf. If you are working remotely, you work. If you are alive, you eat. If you live nearby, you might commute. If you are curious, you visit museums. If you're trying to stay fit, you exercise. One way or another, you can do whatever you feel like. You have time, and because nobody places any demands on you (in deference to your ongoing courageous battle with cancer), the sense of freedom is intoxicating. There are also some new options to consider, unique to this situation.

Wednesday Lunches

This is the free lunch referred to earlier, but it is more than that. It is a well-orchestrated event for proton patients, families, and friends, led by Florida Proton's very own social director, restaurant connoisseur, and master of ceremonies, who also happens to be a licensed radiation therapist (his former position at UFPTI) and the official Patient Services Coordinator. I'll call him Eddie. I'm not sure why, but it fits. Ed Sullivan? Eddie Fisher? Eddie Izzard?

The lunch is held at noon every Wednesday at the Institute on the second floor in a large gymnasium-type room. There is even some random exercise equipment scattered about, with lots of long tables and stacking chairs. Comfortable enough, but not elegant. It's somewhat like an old high school cafeteria setup, but the food is much better, catered by local restaurants, and the portions are generous. It is a well-attended event, which (be forewarned) leads to parking difficulty on Wednesday mornings, even for patients there for treatment rather than lunch. The small private gated lot in front of the Institute will be full early in the day. There is other free parking nearby, but you may have to walk a block or two instead of the usual thirty paces. Don't worry; you can probably do it, but if not, the security guard will gladly allow you to park curbside close to the front door. Just ask. They are all very helpful.

Because UFPTI's clientele includes mostly prostate cancer patients, so do the lunches, but guests will also include child patients and their families, so these affairs are rated G, or at least no worse than PG. Once everyone has their food and is seated, Eddie will grab his wireless microphone and with a spring in his step, greet everyone and begin the official program. The afternoon often begins with a presentation, sometimes given by one of the resident oncologists conducting research relevant to proton therapy, and the specific topics are always fascinating. This is cutting edge, high-tech stuff. Very cool.

Following the opening presentation and any general announcements Eddie makes, the fun begins as he invites newbies to say a few words to the group. A "newbie" is someone who has just begun or will soon begin therapy, or may be in Jacksonville for Phase 1 or Phase 2. Newbies are generally attending their first Wednesday lunch, and standing up to speak even briefly in front of this large crowd is a bit daunting. I did it, and I have no memory at all of what I said. I just felt that if I was going to make any effort whatsoever to become part of this two-month new life, this was an appropriate time and place to start. So when Eddie pointed around the room saying, "Any newbies? Newbies? Where are you, newbies?" I raised my hand, stood up, took the mike, flapped my jaw and tongue for a few minutes, and sat back down, receiving courteous applause. Okay, now I was involved. Good for me.

When there are no more newbies, Eddie looks for graduates. A graduate is a patient who has just finished therapy, or will finish before the next Wednesday. It is their last Wednesday lunch for at least six months, when they return for a checkup. They are generally relaxed, and possibly still euphoric (see Balloonification, Stage 4), and they know what they're talking about. Been there, done that. They know the staff personally, they know a number other patients—proton brothers—and they are in their element. They have attended several Wednesday lunches, listened to other graduates speak, and now it's their turn. This is their show, their commencement address, an opportunity to impart some insight to the newbies, who are hanging on their every word. You will never find a more captive audience.

Some graduates prepare a few notes for this purpose, to make sure they don't forget to say what they intended, leaving out some jewel of information not to be missed. Some compose songs or write poems. I had notes, and gave a lot of thought to what I would say. I had attended every lunch and had seen past graduates speak before me. They were charming, relaxed, and often quite funny. I wanted to be charming, relaxed, and funny, too. We all wanted to have our five minutes of fame. We all wanted to be Jerry Seinfeld, just for a few moments. Or maybe Bob Hope, or even (for some) Henny Youngman.

My fear was that I would try to be funny, but not be funny, suffering a final blow to my ego from which I might never recover. So as I progressed through my eight weeks of therapy I made notes based on observations I thought might be at least amusing to my proton brethren, if not hilariously funny. Most of those observations are in this book, including **The 6 Stages of Balloonification**, which I first presented in my graduation remarks on March 16, 2011. I believe these observations connected with the group. They seemed as amused by them as I was, and I indeed became Jerry Seinfeld for a few glorious moments. I no longer cared about cancer, I was basking in the laughter and applause, and I then understood what treatment at Florida Proton was really all about. It was about being funny. This was my final exam and I had passed. HOORAY!!!

And now it's time for the finale: Eddie invites the alumni to speak. An alum is a former patient who completed treatments at least six months ago, but usually a year or two, sometimes even longer. They are considered the wise elders of proton therapy. They are no longer prostate cancer *patients*; they are now officially cancer *survivors*. Some of them have achieved legendary status in the proton community. They have what the rest of us have yet to attain: they have perspective. They have nothing to hide, nothing to gain. They speak with confidence, and their words are reassuring. As we listen to them we know that we, too, can achieve such greatness, and will soon become and forever remain members of the exclusive club of prostate cancer survivors, along with our other proton brethren. We are the chosen ones, and we are funny.

BOB Meetings

On alternate Wednesdays, just before lunch and in the same location, there is a more serious meeting for prostate patients only. Just the afflicted men. No wives, no friends. This is the "BOB" meeting, Brotherhood of the Balloon, a phrase coined, I believe, by Bob Marckini. The conversation at this meeting is rated R, and sometimes even X. It is not a family-friendly conversation. It is a no-holds-barred discussion of <u>all</u> of the male bodily functions potentially affected by radiation during and after treatments, what to expect, how to be proactive, what kinds of remedies are available, and how they have worked for the individuals attending the meeting. We can offer each other advice and insight even the doctors cannot, unless they have walked in our shoes. We have firsthand knowledge and are the real experts on the topic of being a prostate cancer patient receiving proton radiation therapy. Want to know about that? Ask us. Ask each other.

Without doing a formal survey, I am willing to claim that nowhere else can you find advice like: "Slather up with Preparation-H before your treatment, even if you don't have hemorrhoidal irritation." Makes sense. When it comes to balloon insertion, the more grease, the better, but I hadn't thought of trying this until it was suggested at a BOB meeting. And where else can you discuss which RT has the best balloon insertion technique? Or what exactly Flomax can do? Or Aleve? Or Cialis? These were the kinds of questions I had during treatments, and the BOB meeting was the best to place to find answers from the real experts.

Tuesday Entertainment

It's not all about protons and cancer at the University of Florida Proton Therapy Institute, and the UFPTI folks do their best to help us remember and experience the finer things in life. On the first Tuesday of each month in the main lobby, we are treated to light hors d'oeuvres and wine (cheap, but still wine). Chairs are rearranged to face the center of the lobby where the grand piano is located, and live entertainment is provided for the better part of an hour. This is a special and much appreciated amenity, indeed. The crackers might not be your favorite, the wine may not be featured in fine restaurants, and the performance may not necessarily be your cup of tea, but somehow they add up to a first-rate experience. Very classy.

Restaurant Outings

The Florida Proton folks also know that while protons are the way to your prostate, food is the way to your heart. But what to do, and where to go? Our host, Eddie, is clearly up to the task of guiding us, and knows the local restaurant scene intimately. Some of us have speculated that he might be part owner of some of the recommended establishments, getting kickbacks, using his position at UFPTI as a front for his secret restaurant empire, and that the Institute itself might not even be a treatment facility at all.

If this sounds a bit too conspiratorial, consider the following. We spend most of our Phase 1, Phase 2 time at Shands' facilities, not Florida Proton. What do we do at UFPTI? We drink a so-called barium solution that tastes like a piña colada. We are interviewed. We sign lots of papers. We meet the "doctor" and our "case manager." We pee. We drink. We take a facility tour led by, you guessed it, our buddy Eddie, who does a lot of talking but shows us conspicuously little. We spend quite a while standing in front of a complex diagram of the so-called cyclotron on an easel in the lobby as Eddie rattles on about their amazing technology, but we are not permitted to see the cyclotron itself, and then we have a discussion in a conference room around a table. We are entertained. We're given lunch. We are the subject of a massive maze of misdirection: color-coding for the gantries, little dressing rooms, hospital gowns, RTs, clicks, clanks, ding-dong bells, balloons, computer monitors, and yes, even the gigantic gantry itself. I mean, who likely built that enormous clothes dryer? Maytag? And there's the so-called proton beam that causes no sensation whatsoever. You feel nothing, and are made to believe that is a positive thing. Very convenient, is it not? And the RTs? Come on. People sliding balloons up my butt for a living are just not going to be quite so young, charming and good looking, are they? These "therapists" are undoubtedly part of the empire, getting a kickback of their own. This is big-time stuff.

Add to this the fact that Eddie organizes a restaurant lunch outing for patients every Tuesday afternoon, and a dinner outing on Thursdays. He puts sign-up sheets in the lobby. Eddie frequently shows up at these events, congratulating everyone for making a wise choice to attend. If he suspects you might not be eating enough or participating in these outings, he will miraculously materialize in the lobby from thin air, suddenly interested in you, urging you, even badgering you, to sign up for the next food event.

But what about the multi-page low-gas diet instructions in the UFPTI information packet? Clearly this is an irrelevant diversion. Within a week of arriving for treatments Eddie had corralled a group of us into a Mexican restaurant just a few blocks from Third and Main. Yes, that's right: Mexican! I was confused and a little worried, to say the least, and ordered a grilled chicken sandwich just to be safe. I also had a little bottle of Mexican beer. I didn't want to be a party pooper.

So, conspiracy? Maybe, maybe not, but … I'm just saying. You be the judge.

Gantry Schedule Status

While staying in Jacksonville for proton therapy, timing is clearly crucial. We want specific treatment times so we can be wherever we planned to be, and do the fun things we planned to do. We are busy people. Restaurant reservations, tee times, museum hours, planetarium shows, and so on. Unfortunately, there is the small detail of the time assigned to us by the RTs for our next treatment, and this is almost totally beyond our control.

It is also sometimes beyond the control of the RTs. This is real life, and unpredictable things happen. Patients take longer than planned, through no fault of their own; equipment malfunctions, although harmless, take time to remedy; software occasionally needs to be restarted; computers must sometimes be rebooted; and so on. A 4:00 pm time slot might become 4:30, 5:00, or even later, which might just cause us to lose a dinner reservation.

Naturally, we are concerned about whether our gantry is operating on schedule or not, and Florida Proton knows and has effectively addressed this. In the lobby, next to the receptionist desk near the check-in scanner, there is a computer monitor displaying the status of the blue, red, and yellow gantries. It shows whether they are on time, X minutes ahead, or X minutes behind. There is even a direct feed in of this information in real time to the Florida Proton website so we can check status from a computer or any mobile device with web access. You can look at the status display right now. Just go to www.floridaproton.org and click the gantry times link.

Unfortunately, much like an airport flight status monitor, the data is not always accurate, so its usefulness is somewhat diminished. It is yet another responsibility of the RTs to update the schedule status of their gantry. But as it was explained to me, this is not their highest priority, and I'm truly glad to hear that.

Nevertheless, watching the status of our gantry is something we all do compulsively. The information is there, and even though it is not necessarily 100% reliable data, we like to watch it. I believe this is a mental defect common to most people. It is what also causes us to check the weather forecast as often as we do. We know it must be taken with a large grain of salt, and we probably shouldn't make critical plans based on the data provided, but it's all we have, so we watch it like hawks.

Conjugal Visits

Many of my proton brothers were accompanied by their wives for the entire treatment period, which was comforting and convenient for them. But my wife Lucy and I both still work full time jobs, and it was not possible for her to stay with me in Jacksonville. In hindsight, this was for the best. Although it would have been great for me, she would have become a basket case, driven slowly insane by virtue of being unable to do anything she would call productive. Her professional and personal to-do lists are longer than this book, and I'm glad she was spared an unnecessary two month hiatus.

However, she did make the five-hour drive to see me on several weekends, which were big events for us both. You see, we like each other. We're best friends, and this separation was definitely cramping our style. If it weren't for being able to see each other daily in lengthy video calls via Skype, the loneliness would have been amplified greatly. In this situation, video calls were vastly superior to what voice-only phone calls would have been, but you can't do everything via a video call, if you get my drift.

I've already done my best to explain my possibly feeble reasons for not returning home before the end of my treatments. Aside from the drive, the thought of being home and leaving again, and again, and again felt like more emotional wrenching than I needed at the time. But thankfully, Lucy came to visit several times, momentous events for me. In addition to having the companionship of my best friend, her weekend trips were also clearly conjugal visits.

During the eight weeks of radiation treatments it was important for me to test and monitor the equipment—my equipment. I was able to do a fine job of keeping tabs on peeing and pooping on my own, but the third leg of the stool—poking—was best done with help. So Lucy's visits were very much perceived as critical conjugal visits, especially in light of the "use it or lose it" advice often given. I did not want to lose it, and was happy to use it.

As it turned out, I had not lost it, but under these circumstances my performance anxiety meter was off the scale, so this was certainly not the best sex of our lives. But it did have the benefit of making it clear that further analysis was required, so we experimented a lot during Lucy's visits, and continue to do so now that we're back home. It's important to test this function frequently. Yes indeed.

I must also confess that in addition to cranberry pills, Aleve, and a prescription for Flomax, Dr. Candor offered me a prescription for Cialis if I wanted it, and I accepted the script just in case. I will admit to being a victim of the constant barrage of ads for this and similar drugs. Four hours, blah blah blah. Now, Lucy and I were not having problems, but I can't say with honesty that my performance at sixty is what it was at fifty, forty, or thirty. Which is fine. But then, I had this prescription burning a hole in my pocket, and was becoming curiouser and curiouser, and it finally got the better of me. After watching the prescription collect dust for a few months, I finally caved. I filled it[8], and looking at one of these odd shaped

---

[8] Six tablets per month are all insurance would cover. Are we rationing sex now?

20 mg. pills, I was in awe. This tiny little nothing of a pill was supposed to have the power to do what? So I did my best to cut one into thirds, rather unevenly as it turned out. And then I took the smallest of the three morsels. I waited, and waited, and nothing happened. But then later, when Lucy and I were enjoying each other's company, the little speck of dust kicked into gear right on cue. That stuff works, or at least it works for me.

In case you were wondering.

My Progress Chart

Two months. Thirty-nine weekday treatments. A long, long time. I frequently heard that "it goes by fast" and "it's over before you know it," but that was not happening for me. After a few days it felt like a life sentence. That was partly the result of my own psychological readjustment to and acceptance of a "new normal," but still, that's how it felt. Like I'd be there forever.

I needed a way to mark time, like hash marks on a prison wall, I suppose (forgive the crude comparison). After my third treatment another proton guy told said to me, "Well, Ron, I'm ten percent done!" And although that's not much, it was measurable and seemed like a reasonable milestone. One down, nine to go, instead of one down, thirty-eight to go. Much better. So I made myself a chart on a sheet of Office Depot lined paper. It was ten rows of four squares each—a grid of forty boxes. Along the right margin outside the boxes I wrote 10%, 20%, 30%, etc. so completion of each row—only four treatments—meant another ten percent complete. As soon as I returned from my treatment each day, I shaded another box green. In just a few days there was a fair amount of green, and this way of marking time seemed to help speed things along for me.

Time does move faster on the downhill slope of the hill. Once I finished number twenty, and had only nineteen remaining, the acceleration picked up steam. The light at the end of the tunnel was becoming brighter and brighter, and before I knew it, I was figuring out what had to be done to wrap things up. I was finally able to focus on returning home, for good.

If this is an issue for you, make a chart. Or make marks on the wall (but not at Third and Main).

PROTON TREATMENTS

1	2	3	4	10%
5	6	7	8	20%
9	10	11	12	30%
13	14	15	16	40%
17	18	19	20	50%
21	22	23	24	60%
25	26	27	28	70%
29	30	31	32	80%
33	34	35	36	90%
37	38	39		100%

Treatments with a Twist

Thirty-nine times, not counting simulation. Empty, drink, wait, climb up, roll over, grit your teeth, roll back, don't move, roll over, climb down. Same drill each time. How memorable can any particular treatment be?

Naturally, the first treatment is memorable, and I have already described mine in detail. Nothing quite compares to the first time you experience something new, and at least for me, this drill was new. The final treatment was also notable, but I'm not going to tell you any more about it than I already have. In case you may soon walk this path, I don't want to spoil the surprises that await you at your finale. But don't worry, it's all good.

Treatment #10 was notable for me in that it was the first one during which the balloon insertion was totally comfortable. So much so, that I complimented that therapist afterward, shaking his hand, congratulating him on a fine job, the best so far. Unfortunately, it is considered inappropriate to tip the RTs, and there is no "How'd we do?" customer satisfaction card to fill out and send anonymously to management. So I can only say that wherever you are, RT from my treatment #10, thanks again!

The very next treatment (#11) was also unique, at least up to that point. First, I had a call from a blue gantry RT asking if I could be treated early, at 1:00. They were ahead of schedule (I guess those balloons were slippin' and slidin' smoothly that morning). I was only five minutes away at Third and Main, so I accepted, went immediately to the Institute, emptied, drank, and waited. Ooops. They were not as far ahead as they thought. Another RT sheepishly approached me in the lobby and instructed me to empty and drink again. "Yeah, sorry. I know. Oh well. Do the best you can." RTs are human, after all, and perfection in scheduling something with so many variables is humanly impossible. So, empty and drink again.

This might not sound like a big deal to you, but the problem lies with emptying. We're not always sure we have completely emptied, so having just downed fifteen ounces of water, holding it for quite a while, and being asked to empty and drink again, well, I just wasn't sure I might not end up holding twenty ounces of water, or more. So I peed my heart out, drank again, and hoped I wouldn't have to hold on for too long.

I waited, was retrieved by an RT, and began the usual process: climb up, roll over, grit teeth, roll back ... and that's when their gantry software froze. Nobody's fault. This is technology, right? Stuff happens, and it's reassuring that when it does, everyone knows exactly what to do. When the software locks up (as any software inevitably does), they have to reboot their computer, even when treating an I.T. guy like me. I had no idea how long a reboot required, but I did know I had a full bladder and was beginning to wonder if this would be my day to pee in my pod. Fortunately, the delay was only about fifteen minutes, and I did not embarrass myself. In fact, I was proud of myself. I was becoming rather skilled at this, even in adverse conditions.

Treatments continued and were uneventful until #25, which occurred on a Monday morning. I requested and was given an early morning time slot to ensure that I could drive my daughter Jessica to the airport on time later that morning, after my treatment. She had arrived the prior Saturday, and was the only other extended weekend visitor I had in Jacksonville other than Lucy on three occasions. Jessica's boyfriend (now her fiancé) Reed was in Orlando for a business conference, and I was extremely flattered and touched that he drove from there late Saturday night to spend Sunday with me and Jessica, just to turn around and drive back to Orlando that night. What an attraction I must have been to warrant his going to so much trouble to see me. Or wait, maybe it was to see Jessica. Whatever. I prefer to flatter myself.

So why was treatment #25 notable? Because Jessica accompanied me and took pictures. I was surprised and pleased to find the RTs open to this, and even willing to pose for her. Now, in case you're concerned, I can assure you that Jessica did not photograph any of the most intimate parts of my treatment. That is a bond I share only with the RTs. But still, it was kind of bizarre having my daughter witnessing and recording any of this. And so #25 goes down in history.

Perhaps most memorable was treatment #27. All was going well until I was swung around into the gantry. Then I waited a bit before I was told there would be a delay. As it turned out, there was a system issue that apparently could take as few as five or as many as forty-five minutes to remedy, so they swung me back around out of the gantry, into the room, and posed the $64,000 question: would I like to wait, or have them remove the balloon and start over when the system is ready?

The balloon was not particularly uncomfortable once lodged in the area of my rectum that by then had probably permanently conformed to the exact shape of the familiar balloon, so my first inclination was to wait. It was the insertion and removal that were less agreeable, and I was eager to avoid a repeat performance of that. But the RT became less certain that the system would be ready momentarily, and convinced me to let them remove the balloon. So out it came.

I was then allowed to empty, and they led me back to the dressing room. I was given the option to get dressed and return to the lobby, but I felt that with a foot in the door I didn't want to return all the way to square one. So I asked for a chair that would be more comfortable for an extended stay than the built-in bench, and they wheeled in a standard secretarial office chair for me. There I sat in my gown, reading my Kindle, chatting with an RT, biding time.

Now the trick became identifying the moment the system would be back online forty-five minutes before it happened, because that's when I would have to empty/drink again to be ready for the beam. This was no easy task. I learned that the entire system had shut down. All three gantries were temporarily idle, and the equipment maintenance experts were on the scene, running cables and doing their best to bring the system back online as quickly and efficiently as possible. From the dressing room I had a ringside seat for this performance. And even as I admired the professionalism with which this event was being handled, and as thankful as I was for the advent of proton radiation and all the associated built-in safety mechanisms that protect me when technology hits a speed bump, at that moment what I wanted most was a crystal ball to predict precisely when to drink.

Finally, the RT had a sense that we might be within forty-five minutes of a green light, so I emptied, drank, and returned to the dressing room and my Kindle. Time passed; still no go. Maybe in another forty-five minutes? Sure. Maybe. Probably. Empty, drink for the third time, and read some more. This time they were ready for me, and I found out what it's like to have a double-balloon day. I later learned that it is a rare badge of honor, and makes a great story when I get together with my proton buddies.

The remainder of #27 was uneventful, but these couple of hours are my claim to fame, my bonus balloon day. That would bring my total to forty-one balloons, thirty-nine, plus one in simulation, plus the bonus balloon (no extra charge). To be fair, I have a friend who was given mild chemotherapy along with proton radiation, and to safely reduce his radiation dose per treatment they divided his total over forty-four blasts, making him a forty-five balloon guy. I don't know if he had any bonus balloons, but either way, he wins.

The 3 P's: Pee, Poop, & Poke

Other than curing our cancer, for us prostate cancer guys there are three bodily functions we forever after will monitor closely: how we pee, poop, and poke. Our performance in these areas could well be considered the Prostate Cancer Triathlon. Any prostate cancer treatment can wreak havoc with these, but with proton beam therapy we have high expectations that all three will work pretty well afterwards. Nevertheless, these 3 P's will remain in a constant state of scrutiny to confirm that they are measuring up.

Gone are the days when these activities are mindless, natural, automatic acts. For most of our lives, and certainly for most guys, these regular (or at least semi-regular) activities are just like walking or riding a bicycle: you just do it, you don't think about it. For prostate cancer guys (and yes, maybe some non-prostate-cancer guys aging normally), you not only think about it, you evaluate and score each effort, every time. It's not that we want to. We just do. It just happens that way.

How do we score such things? I've observed the spontaneous emergence of a checklist for each, which might be loosely compared to a Netflix-like 5-star movie rating system. But the criteria for earning stars in our checklists are much more specific and detailed than Netflix's simpler system in which five stars means "loved it" and one star means "hated it." After all, we're not rating movies.

Remember, I did not make these up. They made themselves up. These scales just emerge, taking over like a popup window in your browser that can't be closed. When I pee, poop, or poke, I assign a rating. Don't mean to, just do.

Let's start with peeing.

The Pee Scale

Each of the following items is worth one star, for a maximum of five stars, just like Netflix. A five-star pee is always worth celebrating. If you should happen to hear a guy shouting, "Woo Hoo!" after completing a pee in a public urinal, you might reasonably suspect he is a prostate cancer survivor, and ask him about it after you congratulate him for a job well done.

On the other end of the scale, it is possible to rate a pee event with zero stars, which you cannot do with Netflix. So once again, our scale is better.

★ Was it fast off the starting blocks?

Another way of asking this is, how long did you have to stand there staring blankly at the wall (or, if at a public urinal, probably reading yesterday's sports page) before the first drop graced you with its presence? A quick start, defined as commencing within just a few seconds of hearing the starting gun, earns a star for this category.

★ Was the stream strong?

A slow, endless dribble will slowly drain away your life. Add up all the time you spend standing around waiting for your bladder to empty, and this alone could effectively shorten your life by years. A strong stream, sometimes crudely referred to as "peeing like a racehorse," is also sometimes interpreted (mistakenly) as a sign of manliness. On a visceral level, I particularly enjoy the deep, penetrating sound of a strong urine stream hitting the water dead center at the bull's-eye, don't you?

There is another reason this and the previous star matter. Combined, they determine how long you need to stand at the urinal, start to finish. Who cares, you might ask? When there is only one urinal and other guys are lining up behind you, it becomes more and more difficult to pee. I don't know why it does, it just does. Or when there are two or more urinals and other guys arrive and leave, arrive and leave, arrive and leave while you endlessly continue your feeble effort, you begin to wonder if you should have packed an overnight bag, or maybe post a sign on your back saying, "This lane closed." If you've experienced this, I do have a suggestion that's worked successfully for me: each time someone new arrives, pretend you have just started by making some audible zipper noises, re-executing the usual initial steps, making it look like you too have just arrived and are just getting started. They'll never know you've already been there for your entire coffee break.

★ Did you completely empty your bladder?

I'm still not sure exactly how to determine this. Unfortunately, we have no depth gauge or dip stick that conveniently shows bladder fullness. The only way to guess at this is by noticing how soon it is before you must return for your next effort, and that is the key to understanding the importance of this star. We don't want to pee at every tree. We prefer to pee once and be done with it, at least for the foreseeable future. We want to check it off of our to-do list. We don't want to make a career out of it.

★ Was it painless?

This one is self-explanatory. Nobody likes pain, especially while urinating, which is advertised as a pain-free activity. Prostate guys have a whole new repertoire of possible types of pain while peeing, and we need to make sure it is not due to a urinary tract infection. It might just be irritation of the urethra or something else that will self-correct, but pain is a bad sign, definitely worth a trip to the doctor, and a lack thereof is worth a star.

★ Was there a photo finish?

When you're done, you should be completely done. A couple of shakes and you're outa there. No drip drip dripping endlessly, no squirt squirt squirting, forever waiting for the last splash. Just get it over with, and move on. Life is short, and after all, you might be back again sooner than you think.

The Poop Scale

The star system for pooping is quite different than for peeing, and involves only a four-star scale. Typically, the duration is unimportant. Unlike peeing, you might even consider longer to be better. Bring a newspaper along and this becomes a convenient time to catch up on what's happening in the world. In fact, sometimes an extended poop session can be a welcome, pleasant retreat. But the Poop Scale has other points of concern, again each worth one star.

★ Was it not too hard, not too soft, but just right?

No, this is not the story of the <u>Goldilocks and the Three Bears</u>, but we all know what "just right" is. There is an acceptable range halfway between rock hard and sludge. The further from each extreme, the better, until you get too close to the other extreme. The consistency of Dairy Queen ice cream is not bad, but that's as soft as it should get. On the other hand (don't take that literally), the hardness of day-old Silly Putty is okay, but southern red clay is over the line. We're looking for the hump in the middle of the bell curve on this in order to earn a star for texture.

★ Was it nicely shaped?

I'll bet you've never thought about this consciously, but on a subconscious level you know. Long, winding, snakelike curling is the right ticket. I learned this officially on TV from Dr. Oz. It should naturally coil itself like a garden snake. Cannonballs are intuitively undesirable, and no one wants wormy little wimpy pencil length, random shots. We know what we want without learning it in school. The right shape, the healthy shape, just looks, well … right, and healthy. Worth a star.

★ Was it blood-free?

We generally don't want to see any blood in our stool[9], as it's often called, and a bloodless poop deserves a star. However, you'll have to make a judgment call about whether to award yourself a star for bloodlessness. Prostate patients having undergone proton therapy sometimes do produce some blood, typically in the second year after

---

[9] A "stool," of course, is a small piece of furniture to sit or stand on. To avoid confusion, "poop" is the correct term to use in a medical context.

completion, but this is often considered normal and even a positive sign. It can represent the shedding of old tissue that has gradually been replaced by new, healthy tissue in the rectum, so it may actually be okay, and might even be welcome news. But if vampires begin knocking on your door during your midnight poop, you should probably see a doctor and forgo the star.

★   Was it painless?

Again, self-explanatory. This partly relates to the first two stars (texture and shape): pooping a brick hurts, and squirting sludge can burn. Neither is desirable, and you lose the star. But most importantly, pain can be caused by other problems, and I don't just mean hemorrhoids. Any kind of a tissue tear, lesion, or irritation might cause pain as well as blood, and if you have a lot of pain, well, sorry. You have earned a trip to the doctor, but no star.

The Poke Scale

Okay, I'll tell you, just in case you haven't figured it out. Poking refers to sexual relations. And by that I don't mean third base, I mean home runs. This is the one of the three activities many of us rated frequently even before proton therapy or prostate cancer. Performance is paramount, and is even more closely scrutinized after treatment.

Arguably, this one of the P's doesn't matter much. While we can't survive without peeing or pooping, life can continue with nary a poke. It's just that we don't usually want that, so it does matter, and deserves to be rated. So how do we rate each effort?

This is a sensitive issue, having the potential to change the rating for this book from PG to R, X, or maybe even XXX. To avoid that, I'm going to address this section by using an automobile analogy. Most of you will have no trouble making the appropriate associations. If you do, send me an email and I'll be happy to help you connect the dots. So, here is the rating system for the Poke Scale, a.k.a., the Car Scale.

★ Do you want to get into the car?

Regardless of how well you drive, you can have a star for desire as long as you are interested in taking a road trip. If you have no interest at all in driving, then your total score for this scale is zero and you can ignore the remaining stars.

A diminished interest in driving can happen to anyone for a variety of reasons, and is nothing to be ashamed of. For example, it can be a natural consequence of age; as we grow older, we sometimes just don't think about taking the car out for a spin as often, and that's okay. On the other hand, if you have lost interest in driving and this bothers you, by all means see your mechanic. There might be remedies unknown to you, but worth trying, including dietary, medicinal, or other solutions that can increase your desire to drive.

★ Can you start the car?

If it cranks, you have cleared the next hurdle and deserve a star. While this is no guarantee that you will have a successful trip, it is obviously the necessary first step. If the engine won't crank, you're going nowhere. Now, it's perfectly fine, even highly desirable, to have help with this step. You can turn the key and start the engine yourself, but it can be a plus if someone you love plays a part in this. As it turns out, there are a variety of enjoyable ways to accomplish this, some done independently, others with help. Either way, if you can start the pistons firing, you can have a star.

Related to this is the widely referenced issue of performance anxiety, the concern that no matter how hard you try to start the car, it might just refuse to cooperate. This sometimes becomes a self-fulfilling prophecy, making matters worse, ultimately having an impact on the previous star; if the car never starts, you might eventually lose interest in turning the key. There are several possible solutions to this, and again, your mechanic may have some additional ideas. One that has worked for me is to assign the job of starting the car to someone else (Lucy), thus transferring the responsibility and therefore much of the anxiety to that person. Granted, this approach is not particularly fair, and may not be especially nice, but it can often result in some stimulating, fun strategizing and experimenting in merely making the effort to crank the engine, an effort which can be enjoyable in its own right. If you allow yourself to relax into this approach, you might be pleasantly surprised when the engine sometimes suddenly starts, breaking through this annoying barrier to a rewarding road trip, and earning you a star.

★ Do you have enough gas to complete the trip?

If the car starts, hit the road. You are about to begin an exciting journey. If you're twenty years old, you might be hoping to make a cross-country trip. If you're sixty, you might be satisfied to drive to the corner drugstore (I just hate how many things seem to be age-dependent). Either way, you can have a star if there is sufficient gas in the tank to reach your unique destination, wherever it may be. You do not receive extra credit for making a long trip; you earn full credit for arriving where you intended to go, for making a drive of sufficient duration to feel that it was a pleasant ride.

If you run out of gas along the way, then you cannot have this star. However, keep in mind that there are ways to help ensure you don't run out of gas, and amazingly, some of them are merely mind over matter. You might be able to *think* more gas into your tank if you're sufficiently clever, but if not, see your friendly mechanic. He might be willing to give you some nifty little funny shaped additives that can prolong your journey (but not for more than four hours). Even if you were only planning a short trip around the block, these additives can sometimes provide enough gas to at least get you to the next county, and a longer trip might be quite enjoyable now and then (especially for a *man of my age*).

★ Was there a celebration when you arrived?

Reaching your destination is fine, and sometimes completely sufficient, but you can have one more star if you were greeted with glorious fireworks, a band playing your favorite music, and possibly a high-tech laser light show to punctuate your arrival.[10] While a pleasant journey is a goal in and of itself, thus earning you the previous star, there can understandably be a little letdown if you finish the trip with no fanfare. But if that happens, don't let it negate the fun you had on the way. You can simply say, "Oh, well, we made it to the bandstand, but there's no show today. I guess we'll have to check back another time soon."

In a bizarre twist, you might arrive to find the bandstand buzzing with activity as your arrival celebration is about to begin, but you intentionally pass it by, driving around the block once more because you are enjoying the ride and don't want to stop just yet. This runs the risk of missing the show on your next approach, having to forgo the fireworks that would have been there for you had you stopped earlier, but it can sometimes be a fair exchange leaving you very satisfied. Furthermore, losing this star now can be a blessing in disguise, giving you a perfect excuse to make another road trip soon, anticipating fireworks then. Nevertheless, it means you do not get the star this time.

Hopefully, you will not find the bandstand permanently closed. Hopefully, you will find it open at least some of the time. And given the opportunity, you will no doubt want to stop for the celebration much of the time. After all, you will want to earn this star at least sometimes.

---

[10] If you are a young reader, you might be confused by the separation of completing the trip and seeing fireworks into two distinct star categories. One of my daughters pointed out that in her universe there is a one-to-one correspondence between the two; no arrivals lack fireworks. Furthermore, for the youngest active drivers it is not unusual to have fireworks almost as soon as you get in the car, without completing a trip to even the next corner. This misconception that all arrivals include fireworks is understandable. The men with whom my daughter has driven are in her age bracket, and are not men of my age. She will learn later that you can indeed reach the finish line with great satisfaction, possibly after a very pleasant extended trip, and then happily slow to a gradual halt with no further fanfare.

★ Are you fertile?

I'm ditching the automobile analogy for this one. For most prostate cancer guys, this star is not relevant and does not count for or against you. If you earned all of the prior stars, you have a perfect score. With the exception of a few geezers of questionable sanity, men needing treatment for prostate cancer tend to be old enough to have no interest in further procreation. But prostate cancer engages in age preference, not age discrimination, and there are some younger men who must be treated. Understandably, they might feel slighted without awarding an optional star for continuing to produce aggressive, potent little swimmers even after radiation. This is not always possible, but if you want more kids and can still make some, you can have a bonus star. Fair enough?

Fringe Benefits

If you have not figured out for yourself that prostate cancer (once treated) has benefits, let me clue you in: it does, and you might as well take advantage of them. I mean, come on, guy, you had *cancer*, and you might as well milk it for all it's worth. These benefits are not necessarily huge, but we take what we can get, right?

Looking Good

I have worked for the same employer in the same department for almost ten years, and no one had ever commented on how I look. But since I've returned from Jacksonville it is commonplace for coworkers to approach me, smile, and say with an approving nod, "Hey, Ron, you look good!" Well, maybe I do, or maybe I don't, but I certainly don't think I look much different than I did before cancer or protons. I dress the same, my weight is the same, my height is the same, and the amount of hair on my head is about what it was, at least for now. But who cares about any of that? I look good today! Yeah, baby!

Low Expectations

But hey, I had *cancer*, and two grueling (*hehehe*) months of radiation therapy, so I have every right to claim a little fatigue. It is true that fatigue can be a temporary side effect of any kind of radiation, which I didn't understand at first in Jacksonville. My weekly interview with the nurse included a question about that, and for a while I found it entertaining. "Who, me? Fatigue? Never!!!" That was true until about the sixth week, when I started running out of gas toward the end of the day.

Although this gradually subsided over the weeks following treatment, I did not feel compelled to broadcast the fact that I was fine. That way, at my convenience I could still tell anyone that "sure, I generally feel fine, but I do tend to feel somewhat fatigued unexpectedly. I am just not running at full steam quite yet. I am doing fairly well considering what I've been through, but you can't really expect me to handle as much as before, now can you?" I should be perceived as heroic merely for going to bat every day, and no one should expect maximum performance from me at work or at home. I had *cancer*, you know. I think I'll take a nap.

No More DREs

Since returning from Jacksonville I have had numerous routine doctor appointments to make sure I continue to be in tip top shape. I had my comprehensive annual physical, during which Dr. Perry had always (in recent memory) performed the dreaded digital rectal exam. But this time he did not even offer a DRE, asking, "What for? Why bother?" Yes sir, I was on board with that! I also had a follow-up visit with Dr. Pee, my urologist, who took the same approach. YAY! He said that as long as my exalted PSA continued downward, or at least not significantly upward, and I had no other problems to report, he had no reason to care how my prostate felt. I suspect at some point one of my many doctors will do another DRE, but until then I can't say I'll miss them.

Testing For ED

Perhaps my favorite fringe benefit relates to the concern about post-radiation ED for prostate patients, which does sometimes happen, but is by no means a foregone conclusion. And with protons, ED is (I believe) less likely than with standard photon radiation. For me, it has been a case of *so far, so good*. But nevertheless, as mentioned previously, we must *use it or lose it*, which necessitates the frequent testing of functionality.

I'm sure you guys have your own repertoire of come-ons to initiate maximum intimacy (i.e., home runs), and so do I, including my newest: "Hey, Lucy, I think maybe we should run an ED test tonight, so how about hitting the sheets a little early?" Another effective one is: "I've just taken a Cialis, and we don't want to waste one of those expensive little guys, do we?" Amazingly, both of these usually work. If you've been treated for prostate cancer, try them, but please substitute the appropriate name for *Lucy*.

More Love

Here I'm talking about the other kind of love, the emotional type we crave from our family and friends. Your children, grandchildren, parents—virtually everyone you know—probably loved you before. But now they will love you even more. They have been reminded that you won't be around forever. Sure, we often say things like: "You know, little Billy, Grandpa won't be around forever," but now the words will have more meaning. We're all going to die, and on some level everyone knows this, but now my family *believes* I'm *really* going to die.[11] Probably not soon, probably not from prostate cancer, and probably not by being mobbed at a book signing event. But hey, I get more love!

Discounts

Everyone loves a discount, and believe it or not, there are cancer discounts, and specifically proton patient discounts, at least in Jacksonville. As arranged by our favorite restaurant mogul and all-around good guy, Florida Proton's very own Eddie, proton patients can stay fit with a discounted membership at the local YMCA. We can also enjoy ten percent off at Uptown Market, the delightful little deli on the ground floor below Third & Main's apartments. On the more upscale side, while in Jacksonville we receive free membership privileges at the posh University Club, located on the top (27th) floor of the Riverplace Tower on the Southbank. I almost missed that one, but was invited by a proton buddy to have a drink there on my last evening in Jacksonville, and I thank him again. It offers a fabulous view not to be missed. There are discounts for admission to museums, and probably other special deals I can't remember. I can't promise any of these will still be offered when it's your turn, but just be aware that we proton patients are privileged in many ways.

Your Trump Card

Having successfully completed treatments for prostate cancer, you are entitled to employ that fact to your advantage whenever it suits you. This is especially useful in the universal never-ending competition for sympathy. There is no denying that you had *cancer*, fought the good fight, and are now a cancer survivor. Whatever complaint anyone else might have, chances are

---

[11] This brings to mind Michael Eisner's shocking revelation at the opening of Disney's Animal Kingdom. He said: "Let us be clear...all the animals here will eventually die, as will all the people who come to see them."

good that cancer is worse. You can humor them by listening to a little moaning and groaning about their pain of a pulled muscle, an ingrown toenail, or a broken bone, and then you can just shrug and grin (like the good doctors do), and sympathize a little if you want, but remind them that their malady is not so bad. After all, they could have had *cancer*. Of course, the sympathy then shifts to you, as it should. So play your trump card whenever you want, and enjoy the attention. You deserve it.

Credentials

If your resumé and/or personal bio were lacking, you now have at least one strong credential: you are a prostate cancer survivor who completed proton beam therapy. What can you do with this credential? Well, for starters, you can write a book. As you probably know, prostate cancer books are always in high demand and continually dominate Amazon's bestseller list. We can never have too many books on that topic, now can we?

And in case you happen to think we don't need another book because I have answered every question on that topic, you would be mistaken, as you'll see in the next chapter.

Lingering Questions

If you are thinking about writing your own prostate cancer proton beam therapy book, please include answers to the following questions. Yes, I am providing you with material for your book at no charge, because I will sleep better at night if I have answers to these burning questions:

? How do they decide who inserts the balloon?

Radiation therapists generally work in teams of three in each gantry, but it only takes one of them to insert the balloon. One to insert it, another to remove it, and the third to stand by smiling, nodding approval—a spare RT. Do they consider balloon insertion a privilege, competing to be the one to do the honors? Or is it regarded as the booby prize? Either way, how is it decided each time? It can't be settled by a coin toss; there are no three-sided coins. I suppose it could be done with the long (or short) straw routine. My best guess is they use rock, paper, scissors, a method commonly used for deciding issues of such major importance. But I don't know for sure.

? How many radiation therapists are there at Florida Proton?

On my first treatment day I met my team of three RTs, and I was determined to find out and remember their names. This seemed only right. After all, we were going to be spending time with each other every day, and if we were to intimately bond as I expected we must, I'd want to know their names. This was not Waffle House, and *excuse me, Miss* or *pardon me, Sir* seemed lame. So I asked their names, rolled them around in my mind over and over (I did not have a notepad or pen handy at that moment), and used them out loud for reinforcement. I fully expected to greet every one of them by name the next day, as if we were old pals.

I'll spare you the day by day unfolding of this saga. Suffice it to say that as it turned out, these three RTs were not really my team. I had more than a team; I had an entire village. There seemed to be one or more new players almost daily. A steady stream of new RTs, coming from who knows where. I was constantly introducing myself, shaking hands, learning new names, rolling them around in my head, practicing them out loud, only to find I could not use those names the next day. There were more names to learn, more RTs to meet, more, more, more. ... Where were they all coming from? How many were there? And why so many?

My past therapists were not completely disappearing, just disappearing from me. At various times of day, I was able to spot most of them floating around the building, maybe as someone else's RT of the day. Some even waved at me with a smile. Yes! We do know each other. We do have a past together. Yes! I remember his name!

For a while I held out hope that there would be at least some RTs recycling to me, and I was pleased when that did happen. But there was always someone new showing up. Always yet another RT's name to learn. And so I wondered then, and continue to wonder now: where do they all come from, and how many are there? Where do they keep this seemingly endless stash of RTs?

If I should ever have trouble sleeping at night, I could count RTs instead of sheep, never repeating the same one.

? How do I know if I've emptied?

The doctors and nurses frequently ask us whether we are able to completely empty our bladder. Can you completely empty yours? How would you even know? Does a little bell go "ding" at the end? Does a key part of your body change color? Does your nose twitch? Do you have some kind of a sixth sense? Does the toilet or urinal have an auto-detect device that initiates a flush when it senses completion? Can you tell by a retinal scan? By comparing your weight before and after? How exactly is bladder emptiness identified?

They expect me to know this, but when I ask a doctor or nurse how I'm supposed to tell, they certainly don't know and are not much help. "If you have to go again soon, then it probably wasn't empty before." Well now, that's certainly scientific and helpful, isn't it? Could it possibly be that if I pee now, and pee again in fifteen minutes, the reason is that I have overactive kidneys, that I manufactured enough additional urine in those minutes to prepare me for another successful go at it? Or maybe I just drink so much coffee, soda, and water that I could probably stand at a urinal peeing continuously for the rest of my life, never quite keeping up with my intake of liquids, never emptying my ever-filling magic pitcher of a bladder.

I'll be happy to tell you if my bladder is empty. Just tell me how to figure it out.

? Which is stationery: the gantry or the room?

Okay, of course I know the room and the treatment table are stationary, while the gantry (the dryer drum) rotates around me. I ask this lingering question on behalf of my confused brain, which was unable to accept this simple fact of reality. With the table suspended in the gantry, and me lying on my back, I could only effectively look directly upward at the curved wall of the gantry. I could not see into the treatment room by looking toward my feet. The angle wasn't right. My visual world was reduced to me, my table, the gantry drum, and the proton gun protruding from the gantry wall.

I knew when the gantry movement began because I could see, at least peripherally, that the proton gun's position was changing relative to me. But despite all my pleading with my brain, it would not let me perceive the gantry and the ray gun as moving, with me and my table remaining still. It felt like the exact opposite, an optical or maybe cerebral illusion of giant proportion, similar to two side-by-side trains passing each other in opposite directions. Which train is moving, or could it be both? I knew what was actually happening, but my brain would not accept it. It didn't matter if I focused on a screw in the gantry, as some suggested; that did not work. I tried everything. I really, really tried, but I failed every time, and it was driving me insane.

I finally guessed that I needed more of the treatment room in my field of vision. That was the key. Too much gantry, not enough ceiling/floor. So I asked the RT for a pillow to prop up my head, providing a better viewing angle toward my feet, into the room, and I could see more of it. In this position, my brain short circuited, and started flip-flopping between me moving and the gantry moving, causing some mild vertigo. For brief moments I could stabilize my perception so the gantry alone seemed to be moving, not me, but I could not fully control this. However, in case you find yourself on the table, remember that a pillow under your head and a view of the room from the gantry may be the key to your sanity.

? Will the suntan circles ever be gone?

I neglected to mention earlier that sometime, typically during the last half of treatments, what can be referred to as a suntan circle will appear on each hip at the target point of the proton beam. Remember those magic marker X-marks-the-spots? The radiation gradually produces a pinkish circle about two to three inches in diameter around each X, which looks as if a sunlamp had been focused there. They can itch, although mine never did, and some men use a lotion to relieve the dry itchiness.

These circles are important, because they are the closest thing to actual proof that the proton beam actually does anything. Anyway, it has been quite a while since I finished treatment and my circles have faded a bit, but still remain, so I am wondering: will they be there forever?

? Do the gold markers trigger airport scanners?

This question is no longer a lingering one for me, but it might be for you. I have since had the opportunity to find out whether the gold markers set off alarms when passing through airport security scanners, and apparently (at least so far) they do not. It's a small detail, but I wondered about it and supposed you might wonder, too. Now you don't have to wonder.

If you want the full body pat-down, you'll have to find another way to set off the alarm.

? What if I had not treated the cancer?

After all, I had no symptoms. It is definitely weird to take massively aggressive (and expensive) action to treat a totally invisible problem. Prostate cancer is often slow growing, and many who have it die of something else before they ever even know about the cancer. Would I have been one of those guys? Did I take an unnecessary risk in treating my cancer? If not for my PSA, would I have ever known about my prostate cancer, or cared?

This question will never be answered, of course. My decision to treat it was based on the simple reasoning that I felt certain that the cancer was not going to get better on its own, it might get worse, and although I might outlive it, I might not. So feeling that time could only work against me, and that proton therapy had an excellent outcome profile for prostate cancer when detected and treated early, I took action.

The question of what would have happened had I not acted will linger forever. The only thing I know for certain is that had I not followed the path I did, I would not have written this book, which would have been a terrible tragedy because now I am a cancer survivor and an author!

? How will I feel if an even better treatment option than proton beam therapy is developed?

Someday, possibly in my lifetime, there is always a chance that a more effective therapy for prostate (or any) cancer will be developed. If and when that happens, will I regret what I did? Maybe, but I don't think so. I was diagnosed with prostate cancer at age sixty in the year 2010, and I made the most fully informed decision I could in that context.

My decision in 2010 could not have been based on what I dreamt might become possible in 2030. If a total, simple cure for cancer is available in 2030, I believe I'll be happy to know that receiving proton beam therapy in 2010 allowed me to hang around long enough to hear about 2030's amazing medical advances. But you can't have 2030's cancer treatments in 2010, right?

Nevertheless, how will I feel about it? I don't know, but I suspect I'll be glad for my grandsons in case they end up with prostate cancer. Call me in 2030 and I'll let you know for sure.

Tips for Future UFPTI Prostate Patients

I wouldn't exactly call this advice. It's more like some random, unrelated thoughts you might (or might not) find useful if you're on your way to Jacksonville. These insights are the last dribbles of relevant data escaping from my head with nowhere else to go, and I didn't want them left out.

Learn To Play Golf

Do this before you go to Jacksonville for proton therapy. While there, I discovered that a lot of people play golf. Can you imagine that? It's a slow, silly, boring game, but it becomes the focus of and catalyst for much of the socializing and personal bonding that occurs between prostate guys at Florida Proton. I found other ways to accomplish that, but I will be the first to admit it would have been easier if I were a golfer.

I'm now sixty years old and still don't play, but if I ever have prostate cancer again, the top item on my agenda will be to take some golf lessons before making my first oncologist appointment.

Make Friends

I've heard rumor that making friends comes naturally to a lot of people, but it doesn't to me. I have also heard that sharing the unique experience of receiving protons (and balloons) for prostate cancer would somehow lead to forming lifetime friendships with guys we'd come to think of as our proton brothers (a.k.a., balloon brothers). I was absolutely sure this would not apply to me, and I was okay with that. I would spend my two months at UFPTI, have some cordial exchanges, come home, and forget about it.

But even I—Mr. Antisocial—could not escape this phenomenon, and I did make friends with whom I share that special bond. I even joined the crowd of those who made and carried handy little "proton buddy" business-sized cards, making it easy to swap contact information quickly. Yes, even I became a card carrying proton guy.

So regardless of your tendencies in this regard, I would tell you to let nature take its course in Jacksonville. We proton guys are a surprisingly fabulous bunch of people, and if you're going to become one, I'm sure you'll be fabulous, too! Especially (but not necessarily) if you play golf.

Entertain Your Friends Back Home

While you are in Jacksonville you will probably have countless, "How's it going?" and "How are you doing?" questions from friends and family. It is your responsibility to put them at ease, and this is most effectively done through truth laced with humor.

When you're asked how this radiation thing is working, tell the truth. Tell them the tips of your fingers now glow in the dark. Later, tell them other extremities glow, too. Still later, you can claim to be able to heat a cup of coffee in you bare hands. That you can see through solid brick walls. Light a bulb just by holding it. Change channels without a remote control. Charge your cell phone in your pocket. Pop corn on your lap. Part oceans. Walk on water. Whatever. They don't know, do they? They'll have to believe you, so have some fun.

If they laugh, you'll laugh, and everyone will feel better and have a good time.

Locate Restrooms And Rest Stops

A common post-treatment syndrome for any prostate cancer patient is more frequent urination and possibly greater urgency. Therefore, you should make a habit of beginning each visit anywhere—restaurants, show venues, malls, etc.—by immediately locating the bathroom. Just in case. When it's time to go, it's time to go, and that's not when you want to start researching options.

When traveling by car, start memorizing rest stop locations for the same reason. "Next rest stop 50 miles" is an unwelcome surprise when the next pee stop might unexpectedly be needed in the next five minutes. It's not a bad idea to stop at every opportunity. It's also wise to carry an empty jar or bottle in the car, just in case. I have not yet needed to use mine, but I still keep it in the car. It gives me a sense of security.

As an interesting note on this topic, it is apparently considered inappropriate, undesirable, or maybe even unlawful to pee while traveling on I-26 in Georgia. I surmised this because there are no rest stops heading north, and I believe only one heading south, so pee in South Carolina or Florida, and then race through Georgia as fast as you can. Or stop for a Big Mac, and pee at McDonald's. Just go easy on the Coke.

Consider The Late Time Slots

The early morning (6:00 am or later) treatment time slots are in high demand because once done, you have the rest of the day free (presumably to play golf). But with a late afternoon or evening time slot you still have most of the day free for pleasurable pursuits, so the so-called morning advantage isn't one. Furthermore, there are negatives to early appointments. You give up the freedom to sleep as late as you want, the joy of awakening naturally with the sun—not your alarm clock—and starting your day with a cup or three of smooth, rich, mellow, full-bodied aromatic coffee. Only a fool or an addict (I might be both) fills up on coffee just prior to the *empty, drink, and hold* routine preceding each treatment. Caffeine is counter-productive, making a tough job even harder, and the morning guys have to postpone their first caffeine jolt of the day.

You'll also find that the atmosphere at the Institute is noticeably different in late afternoon or evening, as compared with mornings. The morning crew is friendly as always at UFPTI, but laser-focused on efficiency. They know that when the morning appointments are on time or even ahead of schedule, the afternoons are more likely to be on time, too. So the morning team has a heavy responsibility to set the stage for the rest of the day.

But … and here, with no offense toward anyone in the morning, is my point: the evening is a bit more lively and fun. At least this was true when I was there. The lobby atmosphere is more energized, there's more animated interaction, and it's a much more festive environment. After all, everyone's had their coffee. In the very early morning there is no receptionist (there is no need for one), and that person can set the tone for the entire place.

Also, the therapists for the first appointments of the day don't visit you in the lobby to provide instructions (most morning patients are experienced and no longer need instructions) or to escort you back to the gantry. At that early hour this is usually done by their boss, who is a great guy, a sincere and friendly guy, a dedicated guy, and lots of other superlatives, but … he's not nearly as cute or fun as most of the RTs.

If you've completed treatment at UFPTI, I concede there may be legitimate differing opinions on which time slots are best. I just want to make sure newbies realize that morning, afternoon, and evening times each have their unique advantages.

Eat What You Want

I've already described the preoccupation Florida Proton has with regard to your diet. In the information packet sent to you before you even arrive, they include a multi-paged instruction manual on proper pre-proton dietary restrictions, mostly designed to maintain a low-gas diet. Naturally, newbies become focused on diet, and they are concerned about eating precisely as prescribed. We don't want to sabotage our treatments before we even get there, do we?

Then we arrive, and briefly, the dietary issues are reinforced by our case manager and maybe our doctor. Then along comes Eddie (remember him?), the patient services guy and alleged restaurant mogul. He encourages—even badgers us to sign up for patient outings to restaurants, an alarming number of which feature spicy foods, fried fish, ethnic cuisine, and other clearly counter-productive menus. We begin to wonder, what is going on here?

Let me make it easy for you. The simple answer (in my not-a-medical-expert opinion) is: eat what you want. Just don't let your weight go up or down by more than five pounds. We're told that this could move your prostate, which we definitely want to avoid. And don't eat anything that typically gives you gas or indigestion. Gas can move your prostate, too. For me, beans were off my list in Jacksonville. That's about it. Not complicated.

But obey your doctor, of course. Not me.

Make A Jacksonville Bucket List

Two months is not as long as you think, and Jacksonville has a lot to offer. Despite the seemingly endless tunnel with no light at the end, you will be returning home before you realize it. And you will probably wish you had done some things you just never quite got around to doing. Restaurants, museums, beaches, historical landmarks, farmers' markets, movies, concerts, whatever. I have never used a Segway, those little gyroscopic scooters you may have heard about, and I'd absolutely love to try one. There is a Segway tour available nearby, but I never managed to sign up. A missed opportunity. Maybe next time.

After you've been in Jacksonville for a couple weeks, make your bucket list so you don't miss the chance to do whatever's important to you. Your time there will be over before you know it.

Look Both Ways When Crossing The Street

During my eight weeks in Jacksonville another prostate patient was hit by a bus—literally. I didn't know him, but my understanding is that he was banged up pretty badly and was carried into the gantry on a stretcher each day to complete his therapy. So remember, protons will kill the cancer, but despite the euphoric feeling we often experience after each blast, they will not make you invincible.

Use Skype

Skype is (and if we're lucky, will continue to be) a free service for making video calls. Despite my initial one hundred and fifty percent negative reaction years ago to the seemingly absurd idea that anyone would want to look at me during a phone call, that I would want to be looked at during a call, or that I'd want to look at someone else, I now love Skype. I live in South Carolina, and my mother is a snowbird who migrates between Michigan and Florida. We Skype often, rarely making voice-only calls any more. Skyping really is that much better. It's less like a traditional phone call, and more like an actual visit. So I am able to have such visits with my mother, and with the three of my four out-of-town daughters (I'm hoping the fourth daughter will get on board with Skyping someday soon). I can even see my granddaughter in California, in real time. Very cool.

While in Jacksonville, I Skyped my wife Lucy nearly every night. Seeing her was far more therapeutic than a mere phone call could have been. I Skyped my daughters Caroline, Emily, and Jessica; my mother; and my mother-in-law. If you are a cancer patient your family will want to know how you are doing. They will ask, "How are you doing?" which is a very clever way to seek that information. But no matter how you answer, merely hearing your voice cannot begin to compare with actually seeing you.

Seeing is believing. If you look normal, you are normal. Relatively few people know what to expect from radiation, and would not be surprised to see odd growths sprouting from your head, bloodshot eyes, gyrating limbs, and a loss of hair (protons do not cause hair loss—that would be chemotherapy). Unless I have inadvertently described your normal appearance, having a first-hand look at you is the most reassuring thing anyone can do.

Don't trust me on this, trust my mother, Hecky, who was initially highly skeptical that anything other than "getting it out" with surgery (as my cousin did five years earlier) could cure prostate cancer. Or Laura, my mother-in-law, who had witnessed a horrible, torturous death of a family member from prostate cancer decades ago, and was sure I would be suffering the same inevitable fate in Florida. She seemed truly surprised and relieved to see me healthy and smiling each time we Skyped.

I realized the value of video part way through my treatments, and decided to share the idea with other proton tenants of Third and Main apartments. I bought a cheap webcam for Third and Main's public computer, installed Skype, and invited any tenants interested in seeing a video call to a demonstration. About a dozen or so Skype newbies attended my demo. I had arranged in advance to Skype my California daughter Emily and granddaughter Anneliese. I hauled the big TV screen from my apartment to use in the computer room so their image would be larger than life. It was exciting and fun for everyone, including me.

We then Skyped the teen-aged granddaughter of a couple attending the demo. They had never made a video call, even to their granddaughter, so this was groundbreaking for them. I believe they, and at least a few others of those attending, made the same transition

I did, from, "Who in the world would want video?" to "Who in the world would *not* want video!" Try it and you'll see that a video call is more like a real in-person visit than a phone call. It won't replace phone calls, but it's a better option sometimes, and it was indispensable in Jacksonville.

If you stay at Third and Main, you won't even need your own computer to Skype, assuming my little webcam is still connected to theirs. Otherwise, just bring (or buy, if necessary) your laptop, tablet PC, smartphone, or whatever. Many have a built-in webcam, and Skype (or other comparable services) will probably remain free.

Beware Of PSA Envy

All of us prostate cancer guys are focused like a laser on our PSA, beginning before diagnosis and forever after. Until there are further medical advances, this number (possibly along with an occasional DRE) will remain the quickest and easiest, if not entirely reliable, indicator of our prostate health. So we watch it intently.

But it's more than rational focus, way beyond justifiable normal interest. It borders on obsession. We can recite the history of our PSA dates and numbers from memory. We even know the current score of many of our proton brothers, and we monitor their PSAs as well as our own. Why? Because we care about those guys, of course, and because we have a deep-rooted, genetic, irrational male compulsion to compare our numbers to see whose is better. We need to know our own PSA, but we are driven to know how ours stacks up against theirs.

Our typical greeting to one another is, "Hey buddy, how's your PSA?" Following each new set of lab results we make a mad dash to our computer to notify everyone promptly, knowing they are in perpetual suspense about our latest PSA. Each updated number is big news, eagerly awaited by all. After we complete treatment, our obsession with PSAs becomes apparent even to friends who have not been diagnosed with prostate cancer but are watching their number carefully. Since returning from Jacksonville my office has become PSA Central. Male coworkers regularly stop into my office to report their PSA to me. No kidding. "Hey, Ron, my PSA jumped from 2.5 to 3.6, and I thought you should know." "Well, Ron, my PSA is still holding steady at 3.2, so no biopsy yet for me!" I have become a magnet for PSA news. What we really need is a ticker-tape-like crawler along the bottom of our computer monitors, giving up-to-the-minute data on everyone's PSA at all times, along with the usual stock market updates.

Unlike other male-to-male comparisons in which bigger is better, in this case smaller is better. When I learned that my friend Peter's PSA was 1.1 only three months after completing treatments while mine was 2.1 six months after finishing, I reacted (to myself) with typical male PSA envy. I was jealous and felt it wasn't fair; mine should be less than his. I was somehow less successful, inferior in my performance. The fact that we are unique people, different in countless ways—he has a Ph.D. while I have a B.S., he roots for Alabama while I'm for Michigan, his wife is from South America, mine's from South Carolina, he's retired, I'm not, he's never written a book about protons, prostates or cancer, and I have—seemed irrelevant. His PSA was better than mine. Simply not fair.

Intellectually, I know our PSAs cannot and should not be compared, and I know I can be happy with mine regardless of his. But nevertheless, PSA envy still sometimes occurs. So even if *you* can't completely avoid it, at least now you can be on the lookout for it. When his PSA is better than yours, you can be happy for him, while knowing that your feelings of PSA envy are normal.

Make Yourself Available To Newbies

Once you finish proton beam therapy, you are immediately considered an authority on the topic, as you should be. No one knows better than you (and those reading this book) what's entailed. Newbies or prostate cancer victims considering proton therapy will want to talk with us veterans, and in the spirit of paying it forward, I encourage you to allow your name to be included on Florida Proton's contact list, as mine is. This may be the one circumstance in your life in which you are guaranteed a rapt audience, eager to hear every word you have to say on the topic. You can ramble on and on and they will listen attentively, thanking you profusely for your time, knowledge, and wisdom.

In contrast, see how that works with your wife, and let me know.

Proton Weenies

I'd sincerely like to know what the future holds for me. Can someone please help me with that? Like, how low will my PSA go, will I remain healthy, how long will I live, will I lose much more hair, will <u>PROTONS versus Prostate Cancer: EXPOSED</u> be made into a movie, and if so, who will play the lead role … lots more like that. No?

I'm sixty-one and in reasonably good health. It wouldn't hurt me to lose a few pounds, but I doubt that's going to happen. I should probably do some muscle strengthening exercise in addition to using the elliptical, and there might be a slim chance of that happening. But you know how it is. When things are going pretty well, the drive might not be there, and things are going well enough right now.

Although I am currently a well-oiled marvel of a machine, I do know at some point the parts will start wearing out. And the question arises: as I pass the 100 year old milestone and possibly fall into some disrepair, who should I blame? Fortunately, I've had prostate cancer and that will be my eternal scapegoat for anything negative that occurs hereafter in my life. I am looking forward to a long, blameless life of passing the buck whenever it's convenient. A ready arsenal of phrases like: "This must be because of some lingering effect of that dang radiation years ago," or "Those pesky little protons! What will they cause next?" will help me shift the blame in almost any situation. After all, protons were not only supposed to kill the cancer, but should have fixed *everything*—and with a lifetime guarantee. Well, that's certainly reasonable, isn't it?

There is more truth in this than you might think. We who have completed proton therapy for prostate cancer run the risk of becoming Proton Weenies. We whine and complain about every little bodily function not measuring up to our new superhuman standards. "Help, doctor, please! It took me 12 seconds before I saw a drop of pee pee this morning. What shall I do???" Or maybe: "I ate a normal super-sized meal at the new Mexican fast food restaurant down the road and had the backhouse trots and I just know it's because my rectum is falling apart from protons so I'd better hurry up and post this on the forum and see what the other guys think." Or how about: "What will I do now that the Cialis is only keeping me going for three hours instead of four? I'll see how many brothers have experienced that, too, or maybe I better go to urgent care now!"

I had a few minor complaints when I saw my urologist, Dr. Pee, last week. Guess what: he shrugged (ha) and said: "Let's see now, when is your birthday? Aha! 1950? Well, there you go!" And there I go. I am growing older, and things are going to peter out along the way to some degree or another, and it won't always be because I had prostate cancer or proton beam therapy. It's just the way it works. My grandmother didn't like it. My mother hates it. And I'm pretty sure I won't enjoy the downward slide of the machinery of life much, either. Must be hereditary.

I know I'm going to die (I read that on the Internet). I don't know how or when, but it will probably not be from prostate cancer. I can check that one off my list. In the meantime, I have a new lease on life and plan to make the most of it. I've learned that quality of life is subject to change without notice, and *so far, so good* is as good as it gets, so I better enjoy it now. Thankfully, I have Lucy to enjoy it with, and I don't plan to saddle her with a Proton Weenie for the next fifty years. Just wouldn't be fair.

Uh, oh. Wait a minute. I think I hear someone asking, "How's it going back there, Mr. Nelson?"

Excuse me, please. I'm going to empty and drink.

Appendix A: My Timeline

1950 May 5   Born healthy—no prostate cancer—PSA=0

2004 December 3   First recorded adult PSA=3.0

2007 March 26   PSA=3.8

2008 March 17   PSA=3.7

2008 September 29   PSA=4.5

2008 November 3   PSA=4.4

2009 January 5   PSA=4.2

2009 April 6   First meeting with urologist, including DRE at no extra charge. Prostate felt "firm with good elasticity"—decided to watch and wait.

2009 September 8   PSA=4.8

2009 October 1   Second meeting with urologist—he scratched his head, I scratched mine—we decided to continue active head-scratching.

2010 March 22   PSA=5.1

2010 April 26   PSA=5.1, steady as she goes.

2010 July 1   Third urologist visit—with PSA above 5, we are now more concerned—he suggested PCA3 test, which sounded exciting, so I agreed.

2010 August 16   Urologist administered PCA3 test—way more exciting than expected—urologist is no longer my friend.

2010 September 16	PSA=5.9, PCA3=50% (>35% is positive)—biopsy recommended—I agreed—decided I'd better make urologist my friend again.[12]
2010 October 14	First (and only) biopsy performed—Versed given orally—can't remember a thing, but I'm told I did well and was entertaining.
2010 October 21	**CANCER**—positive biopsy—Stage T2a, Gleason 3+3=6—I began aggressively researching treatment options.
2010 October 23	Broke the news to my family.
2010 November 1	Met with Harold at Barnes & Noble to discuss proton beam therapy, which he completed at the University of Florida Proton Therapy Institute in early 2010.
2010 November 2	Learned from UFPTI that the typical 8-week proton regimen costs $160,000—estimated my home equity and value of collectible guitars for possible sale.
2010 November 3	Mailed application package to UFPTI, to get the ball rolling, just in case.
2010 November 8	Discussed insurance application strategy with UFPTI—decided to delay sale of home, guitar, and children—asked urologist to provide letter of referral and medical necessity for proton beam therapy.
2010 November 22	PSA=5.3—Hey, it's falling—maybe this is all just a mistake.

---

[12] Never allow a biopsy to be performed by a urologist who is not your friend.

2011 November 23	Insurance approval received for proton beam therapy at UFPTI—onward!
2010 December 3	Colonoscopy done—no problems—repeat in 10 years.
2010 December 5	Received instructions from UFPTI—eating is now illegal.
2010 December 6	PSA=5.8—Okay, it's back up—guess it's not a mistake.
2010 December 9	Met with Bob (UFPTI graduate[13]) and his wife in their home—gained more insight into proton therapy versus surgery.
2010 December 14	Made reservations at Third and Main for Phase 1, Phase 2, and Phase 3.
2010 December 16	First trip to Jacksonville (with Lucy) for Phase 1, Phase 2.
2010 December 17	First visit to UFPTI—met with my oncologist and his nurse (my case manager)—did lots of paperwork—paid for my portion (copays) for treatment—had CT scan at Shands Scan Shack.
2010 December 20	Phase 2, Day 1: bone scan and chest X-ray (big Shands building), MRI (Shands Scan Shack)—lots of paperwork, everywhere.
2010 December 21	Phase 2, Day 2: Fleets enema, gold marker placement, more paperwork—UFPTI facility tour.

---

[13] Bob was just days away from having a radical prostatectomy when he first learned about PBT. He canceled his surgery, went to UFPTI, and is doing well.

2010 December 22	Phase 2, Day 3: Simulation at UFPTI—empty, drink, first balloon, CT scan, open MRI, pod creation, magic marker "X" on each hip for laser alignment—spent the rest of the day in the apartment fighting severe allergic reaction to Flagyl.
2010 December 23	Homeward bound!!!
2010 December 24	The first of cascading visits from family for the holidays.
2011 January 2	Family visits conclude.
2011 January 19	Back to Jacksonville (without Lucy).
2011 January 20	Phase 3 begins—first treatment received at UFPTI (not Shands—their part is finished).
2011 January 26	First Wednesday FREE lunch (making sure I get my money's worth).
2011 January 28	First weekend visit from Lucy—hooray!!!
2011 February 1	Entertainment in UFPTI lobby for "First Tuesday" of the month—drank no wine because my treatment was to follow the performance.
2011 February 3	First BOB meeting (alternate Wednesdays)— highly informative—then treatment #11: empty, drink, wait—then repeat: empty, drink, wait—software problems.
2011 February 4	First haircut away from home—possibly more risky than the protons.
2011 February 11	Lucy's second visit—hooray!!!!

2011 February 19	Jessica (daughter) and her boyfriend (now her fiancé) Reed arrived for the weekend—hooray!!!
2011 February 21	Jessica took photos of my treatment—also repeated UFPTI tour with Jessica—saw the simulation room for what seemed like the first time, as I was sick from Flagyl during simulation and not very focused on the room.
2011 February 25	Lucy's third visit—hooray!!!!!!!!!
2011 March 1	Balloon Bonus Day—total system shutdown of all three gantries—empty/drink/wait three times—two balloons—my claim to fame.
2011 March 4	Peeing very slowly—tried Flomax (in addition to the cranberry tablets and Aleve I was already taking daily)—worked great—peeing like a racehorse!
2011 March 5	Lunch visit from my good friend Buren and his son—enjoyed the preteen son's reaction to hearing about the balloon.
2011 March 15	PSA=9.3[14]—YIKES! I knew it could go up—would have preferred down—I wasn't worried.
2011 March 16	FINAL TREATMENT (#39)—spoke as a graduate at Wednesday lunch—introduced **The 6 Stages of Balloonification**, and enjoyed my five minutes in the spotlight.
2011 March 17	HOMEWARD BOUND!!!

---

[14] UFPTI wants an exit PSA as a benchmark for the record, but it usually doesn't have much significance because the prostate is highly irritated at that point from two months of radiation blasting. Many PSAs go down, while some go up.

2011 May 13	Accidentally began writing this book, not realizing that's what I was doing at the time.
2011 June 13	PSA=2.6, my lowest in recorded history!
2011 September 10	Officially acknowledged (to myself and Lucy) that I was writing <u>PROTONS versus Prostate Cancer: EXPOSED</u>.
2011 September 26	PSA=2.1, still heading in the right direction.
2011 October 9	Finished first complete draft of <u>PROTONS versus Prostate Cancer: EXPOSED</u>, handed it over to Lucy for proofreading, and the rest is history.
2011 December 8	PSA=1.3—YES! Apparently that beam has some potency after all.

Appendix B: Glossary of Terms

The following definitions are not necessarily medically or scientifically accurate and should not be used in any way to assist you in making any decision of any kind on any subject in this or any other universe at any time for any reason. These are my definitions and mine alone, and I accept no responsibility whatsoever for their use or misuse.

Accessory
: A derivative of "accessorize," a term commonly used in the fashion world. At UFPTI, your "accessory" is a most unattractive necklace, its only decoration being a plastic pouch containing a business card sized bar-coded identification card and a treatment scheduling card. It is used by patients at the self-check-in station near the reception desk before each treatment, immediately upon arrival.

Balloon
: (1) A festive, multi-colored, air-inflatable, stretchable rubber sack used at parties and other fun occasions as a decoration, or (2) a miserable, mono-colored, saline-inflatable baggie shoved up a prostate patient's butt (often with the aid of a special lubricant) to pull the rectal wall away from the prostate, and to help stabilize the prostate during proton radiation treatment.

Balloonification
: As in "The 6 Stages of Balloonification," refers to the psychological evolution of a proton/prostate patient's relationship with balloons; see Balloon (2).

Biopsy (prostate)	A medical procedure usually performed by a urologist to remove a dozen or more tiny chunks of a man's prostate gland by poking snippy-needles into the prostate through the butt while watching with an ultrasound monitoring system also crammed into the same limited space as the needle mechanism. The ultrasound monitor is necessary to ensure the samples removed are in fact from the prostate and not the heart, liver, stomach, larynx, or other nearby organs. The extracted tissue is then examined in the hope of finding cancerous cells. If such cells are not found, there is no cause for concern; more samples can be taken at a later time, continuing the "snip, look, repeat" process until cancer is found or the prostate has been entirely removed, snip by snip.
BOB	An acronym allegedly coined by prostate cancer survivor and author Bob Marckini, short for Brotherhood of the Balloon, an elite group of fine men who have shared the unique experience of receiving balloons up their butts.
BOB meeting	Meetings on alternate Wednesdays for prostate cancer patients only, where men, under the clever guise of discussing medical issues and sharing useful information, revert to the kind of locker room talk not used since junior high school.

Butt	A portal through which, for prostate patients, more things enter than exit, including gold seeds, suppositories, enemas, Preparation-H, lubricant, fingers, needles, ultrasound scopes, and last but not least, balloons. Things exiting via that doorway include most of the above items, and of course, poop.
Cancer	A constellation in the northern hemisphere between Gemini and Leo.
Case Manager	The nurse assistant to a prostate patient's oncologist, trained to ask with great compassion (never smiling, and especially not smirking) a weekly series of probing questions about urinating and defecating while patients undergo proton beam therapy.
Cialis	One of the few recreational drugs available legally in the United States, for which men will find or create any excuse—even cancer—in order to get some.
Cranberry	A berry used to make delicious fruit juice or tiny, tasteless pills alleged to promote urinary tract health when taken by prostate cancer patients and others with urinary systems.
Cyclotron	A science-fiction-like device which produces protons for use in radiation therapy. Cyclotrons may or may not exist, as no one has ever seen one other than in artists' renderings, and the protons they are presumed to create cannot be seen, smelled, heard, or felt, even while standing directly in their path.

DRE	An acronym for Digital Rectal Exam, a procedure typically involving a doctor, a hand, a glove, a finger, and a butt. And maybe some lubricant.
Flomax	A drug that can make you pee like a racehorse, even if you are not one.
Food	Something prostate cancer patients are not allowed to eat for several weeks before and during proton treatment for fear it might cause weight gain or flatulence at inopportune times.
Gantry	A gigantic structure three stories high, shaped like a huge clothes dryer drum, in which a patient is suspended on a treatment table while various ding-dong sounds, whirring noises, clicks, clanks, and footsteps are heard, and where the illusion of treatment occurs as the drum rotates and the so-called proton beam generated by the so-called cyclotron shoots the patient and invisibly, painlessly kills the cancer in a series of brief daily zaps.
Gold Markers	Tiny bits of gold, about the size of a grain of rice. Four of them are implanted into the prostate to reveal its position via low-level X-rays used during treatments to ensure exact alignment of the prostate. These fiducial markers are gently placed into the prostate in much the same way a biopsy is done, but in this case the urologist is putting something in, and taking nothing out. The markers remain the property of the patient after completion of treatment, and although they are a small investment, they have a high rate of return and have virtually no risk of theft or loss.

Golf	A slow, time-consuming outdoor game involving knocking a tiny ball into a hole in the ground with a stick, used to keep prostate cancer patients from getting into trouble between proton treatments, and as an excuse for making friends.
Oncologist	A medical doctor specializing in the treatment of cancer, relying heavily upon a skilled case manager to conduct nearly all patient interaction, and highly-trained radiation therapists to administer patient treatments with the notable exception of DREs, which most oncologists enjoy handling personally.
PCA3	A simple urine test to help determine whether a prostate biopsy is indicated, involving a urine sample taken after a brief (a minute or so) but torturously enthusiastic and vigorous massage of the prostate into the bladder via the rectum, using the urologist's gloved finger. This is a potentially life-threatening procedure, as several urologist's have been nearly killed immediately afterward by the patient. Fortunately, there have been no reported fatalities to date, and an amicable patient-urologist friendship usually resumes within a few days of the procedure, especially if a biopsy is scheduled.
Photons	Invisible particles commonly referred to as X-rays, most appropriately used as a tool by superheroes in old science-fiction movies, television programs, and comic books to let them see through solid objects.

Pod	A container that, when very small, usually holds between three and five peas, and when much larger, can comfortably hold a full-sized prostate cancer patient.
Protons	Invisible particles created by a cyclotron, often used to kill cancer cells painlessly, while barely touching healthy cells on the way to or from the target, a true miracle of modern science. To the naked eye, protons and photons are nearly indistinguishable, but despite this close resemblance and their nearly identical spelling, they are entirely different, and one should not be mistaken for the other. Also, protons cost way more than photons, but they're worth it.
PSA	An acronym formerly used for Public Service Announcements, but now almost always used to refer to the Prostate Specific Antigen produced exclusively by the prostate gland in men. Measured via a standard blood test, an abnormally high PSA level can indicate prostate cancer, but not necessarily, and a low one might indicate a healthy prostate, but not necessarily, but it's all we have to go on at this time so we obsessively watch it to determine if additional action is warranted. Knowing your PSA number can be the difference between being clueless and having at least one clue, which is all the PSA reading really is. It is also a readily available topic of conversation with your urologist when there is nothing else worthwhile to discuss.

PSA Envy	A common affliction in which men watching their PSA before, during, and after treatment for prostate cancer obsess over how their number compares to that of others. When other men have lower PSA numbers in comparable circumstances, an emotionally charged reaction of intense jealousy occurs, but rarely results in violence.
RT	An abbreviation for Radiation Therapist, a person of either gender, typically no older than 23, extraordinarily good looking, kind, gentle, and competent, having completed several years of formal training in (among other things) the proper insertion and removal of a balloon into and out of a man's butt with or (in extremely rare cases) without sufficient lubrication.
Shands	The nearby group of medical facilities that are not part of, but are used by UFPTI for imaging services—CT scans, MRIs, bone scans, X-rays—all the less cool parts of treatment.
Towel	An absorbent cloth placed on the floor at the base of a urinal to capture stray droplets not quite making it into the receptacle due to the *poor-aim* side effect of many proton/prostate patients during treatment.
Triathlon	This refers to the 3 P's of prostate cancer patients: pee, poop, and poke. Doing well in all three areas after completion of any method of treatment wins this triathlon. Official rating scales are those described in this book.

UFPTI	Acronym for the extraordinarily lengthy name of the excellent proton treatment facility in Jacksonville, Florida: The University of Florida Proton Therapy Institute, also referred to as Florida Proton or simply the Institute.
Urologist	A prostate cancer patient's favorite doctor, trained to discuss PSAs, administer PCA3 tests, perform biopsies, and most notably, give DREs. A urologist's primary responsibilities are to perform DREs, shrug, and grin.
Vanity	A human personality trait commonly found in both women and men, including men with prostate cancer. Interestingly, prostate cancer treatment via proton radiation therapy kills vanity along with the cancer cells, although no formal relationship has been proven to exist.
Versed	Sorry, I can't remember what this is, but I think I like it.
Water	The beverage of choice for most proton-therapy-prostate-patients, who simply cannot seem to get enough of it, nor retain it for long.
Wednesday Lunch	The only part of proton beam therapy at UFPTI that is free, every Wednesday.

Acknowledgements

At the top of the list is Lucy, who has stoically and graciously endured hearing endlessly about, and reading repeatedly about the thrilling topics of prostate cancer and proton beam therapy. I am certain there is no one happier than Lucy that this book project is finished. She was my first, last, and most frequent proofreader, made countless suggestions for improvements in content and style, and I and everyone reading this book owe her a debt of gratitude. May I be blunt? It would have been a very mediocre book without her help. Also, the warrior drawing, the Gleason happy/mean face cancer cells (based on her memory of those drawn by my urologist), and the sketch of my pelvic area were her creations. She is a woman of many talents, but those are the relevant ones I am comfortable sharing with you. From start to finish, her words of encouragement ("Yes, dear, you really have written a nice little book. Keep working on it. It's getting there.") kept me moving steadily forward toward the finish line.

Next to Lucy, no one has scrutinized my manuscript quite like my wonderful daughter Emily, who deserves most of the credit for helping me appear to be literate. In grade school, I depended on Aunt Gilda to proofread my papers in search of unneeded commas; now I depend on Emily. At my request, she mercilessly nit-picked this book to death, phrase by phrase, word by word, comma by comma, until the result was sufficient to give the miraculous illusion that I am a competent writer. The proof is that you made it to this page without accusing me of willfully impersonating an author. However, I stubbornly accepted only about 80% of Emily's corrections; if you do find any errors, they are undoubtedly in the other 20%.

And then there's my brilliant daughter Jessica. That would be Dr. Jessica R. Nelson, Ph.D. to you. I am not a doctor of any kind, but knowing I could produce one allows me to believe I have some intelligent genes. Jessica was an early proofreader, mostly for content rather than grammar, and provided numerous excellent and very critical suggestions, nearly all of which are reflected in the final copy. You'll recall that she also paid me a visit in Jacksonville, spent a wonderful weekend with me, and took the only photographs I have of my experience there. You can thank Jessica for the book cover photo and the gantry picture inside. She says you're welcome.

My friend Harold Mills was also one of a handful of early proofreaders, but more importantly he is the first person with whom I spoke extensively about proton therapy, giving me a wealth of useful information and encouragement. I sincerely thank Harold for that, as well as his friendship. I may as well also thank him for his dual role in my life; he not only survived cancer, but survived teaching AP History to my daughters Emily and Caroline in high school. Someday, Harold, you'll have to tell me which the greater challenge was: teaching them, or treating prostate cancer.

These acknowledgements would be seriously incomplete without thanking my urologist, Dr. Richard Morrow (a.k.a. Dr. Pee), a heck of a nice guy. He is a rare breed of urologist, and one who takes the Hippocratic Oath seriously. He's the kind of guy who will call you at home on a Sunday night to avoid any delay in sharing the excitement of your new low PSA score. If he had not included proton radiation therapy in his list of treatment options to consider, I can't be sure I would have found out about it on my own. I will be forever grateful to him for that, and for knocking me out before my biopsy.

Finally, it is really not possible to express how grateful I am for all the superb medical care and personal attention I received from my local doctors (and now you know them all), and of course from everyone I encountered at the University of Florida Proton Therapy Institute in Jacksonville. From the security guards to the night nurses, from the receptionists to the oncologists, from the intake staff to the radiation therapists, from the physicists to the publicists, this was the embodiment of excellence. I hope you won't, but if you should ever need treatment for cancer you would be extremely fortunate to have a similar experience, and whether you end up in Jacksonville or elsewhere, I wish you nothing less than a UFPTI-caliber encounter.

When you've finished, write a book.

About the Author

Ron Nelson was born and raised in Michigan, graduated from the University of Michigan, moved to South Carolina soon afterward, lived in Charleston for almost twenty years, later moved to the rural midlands near Columbia, and does not play golf. He enjoys peace, quiet, solitude, birds, autumn, building fires, his dog Baxter, high octane fresh ground drip coffee, southern mustard-based barbecue (Maurice's), Netflix, professional tennis, good conversation, and many styles of music, especially finger-picking solo acoustic guitar.

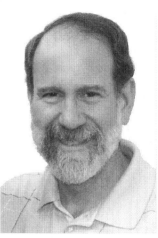

Ron is the helplessly happy husband of Lucy, the proud father of four fantastic daughters (Julie, Jessica, Emily, and Caroline) and the grandfather of three (Anneliese, Ben, and Dorsey) … so far. And he loves and admires his marvelous mother (Hecky).

By day, Ron is the I.T. Training Coordinator for the Information Technology Department of Richland County Government, teaching employees to effectively use their computers. When he is not working or fighting his courageous battle with cancer, he plays guitar, reads his Kindle, and eats whatever he wants, regardless of whether it gives him gas.

* * * * *

Please contact him at **Ron@ProtonsExposed.com**.
He'd love to hear your questions, comments, and stories.

www.ProtonsExposed.com

67889234R00093

Made in the USA
Charleston, SC
27 February 2017